PETS LIVING WITH CANCER:
A PET OWNER'S RESOURCE

PETS LIVING WITH CANCER:
A PET OWNER'S RESOURCE

ROBIN DOWNING, DVM

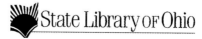

AAHA Press
12575 W. Bayaud Avenue
Lakewood, Colorado 80228

Library of Congress Cataloging-in-Publication Data
Downing, Robin, 1958-
  Living with cancer: a pet owner's resource/Robin Downing.
    p. cm
  Includes bibliographical references and index.
  ISBN 1-58326-022-6
  1. Pets—Diseases. 2. Cancer in animals. 3. Veterinary oncology. I. Title.

SF981.D68 2000
636.089'6994—dc21   00-022489

Contents

Foreword

Cancer. The word is as dark and empty as the disease it defines. A diagnosis of cancer often brings with it feelings of overwhelming fear, a spiraling sense of loss of control, and, most devastating of all, the loss of hope. This occurs regardless of whether the patient is a human family member or a precious pet. When we face the diagnosis of cancer in a beloved pet it is even more difficult, for we must make important and life-changing decisions for creatures that rely totally on our own judgments for their well-being. These precious animals not only share our homes, our lives, and our experiences, but they share our hearts. We have experienced their love as unconditional, and we seek through our own decision-making process to provide for them the quality and dignity of life that we know they deserve. Seeking the most appropriate care for these wonderful friends is the very least we can do as a response to their love and affection. Our goal becomes to share as many possible moments within this wonderful relationship we term "the bond."

The beacon of light one must carry to defeat the darkness of cancer is knowledge. The American Animal Hospital Association and Dr. Robin Downing have taken a bold, important step to conquer the hopelessness of cancer with this book. The information within these pages takes the reader to the first of three steps.

The first step in facing cancer head-on is to dispel the myths of the disease as well as of its treatment. Instead of viewing cancer and cancer therapy through a shroud of myths and misconceptions, the chapters within this book afford us the information we need to chip away at the fears about cancer that are encased within us all and begin to replace them with truth. It is only by dispelling the myths and misperceptions that we can think clearly, make decisions, and begin to find the hope and opportunities that lie before us as we deal with cancer.

The second step of cancer care is as vital as the first. Care of a beloved animal can only be accomplished if it is done as a team. At the center of that team is the person who knows your pet's needs and desires better than anyone else in the world: you! In addition, you must carefully find and entrust your beloved pet to a veterinary health care team. All members of the staff, from the office personnel to the technicians, nurses, and other staff, must understand that they play a vital role in the care of the cancer patient and you and your family. The veterinary health care team must actively incorporate you into this team through education and empowerment to provide ongoing day-to-day care and assessment. Without your input, attention, and care, as well as your ongoing assessment, care of the cancer patient will not be optimal.

Once the caring team is forged to include at least the veterinarian, veterinary health care staff, and caregiver, and we shed ourselves of the misperceptions of cancer, then we can begin to conquer the emotional component of this disease. Once you have stripped away this dark, emotional cloak and, as a caregiver, have built a team around you, the cancer affecting your pet becomes attackable, diagnosable, treatable, manageable, and, in many cases, curable.

At this point, the care may begin. For the cancer patient and the care-giver, this must be *compassionate care*. This is the third and final step. Compassionate care is the single most important operative term in cancer medicine. A response by the veterinary health care team based on an understanding and appreciation of the family-pet-veterinary bond, compassionate care applies science through the heart.

As you and your beloved pet face the uncertainty, the darkness of cancer, I would urge you to break through that dark by dispelling the myths with information and knowledge. This book will be an important guide in helping you begin this process. You must then build a team with your veterinarian, his or her staff, and other experts within the veterinary profession; cancer is a big disease that must not be taken on alone. And finally, seek out compassionate care provided by people that recognize and value the magic you and your pet share. It is then that you and your pet will live daily in the hope and the wonder of that precious relationship we all know, yet find beyond our abilities to explain ... the bond.

Gregory K. Ogilvie, DVM
Diplomate ACVIM (Specialties of Internal Medicine, Oncology)
Professor and Head of Medical Oncology
Department of Clinical Sciences
College of Veterinary Medicine and Biomedical Sciences
Colorado State University
Ft. Collins, Colorado

Acknowledgments

No book like this can come to completion without the input, influence, and impact of many, many individuals. Many incredible people behind the scenes have assisted in one way or another with this project. I want to thank a few of those people here.

My editor, Mary Kay Kozyra, who had the vision to know the time was right for a book such as this. Dr. Steve Withrow and the oncology team at the Colorado State University Veterinary Teaching Hospital, Ft. Collins, who have helped so many of my patients over the years and who gave me the gift of time with my own Murphy. Dr. Greg Ogilvie, also at CSU—my mentor, my colleague, and my friend, who has taught me about marrying the head with the heart, the science with the soul.

Thanks to the many animal patients who have taught me so much through the years about unconditional love and being a more compassionate veterinarian. Many thanks also to the families who have entrusted the care of their beloved animal companions to me and my team.

My greatest thanks belong to the Divine One, for blessings in abundance, and to my life partner, Sharon DeNayer, who has been with me throughout my education and beside me every step along my career path. She is my confidant, anchor, best friend, and most stalwart supporter.

INTRODUCTION

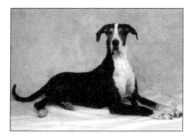

Murphy at age 6 1/2.

❖

The last thing I expected when I agreed to adopt Murphy, a beautiful black and white Great Dane who had been my patient since she was a puppy, was to diagnose bone cancer within a week of bringing her into my home. That day I entered uncharted waters, for though I have always maintained a special interest in oncology, treating cancer patients both within my practice and with the help of veterinary cancer specialists, never had one of my own animal family been afflicted.

Murphy's bone cancer was in her left front leg, just above her wrist joint. On the day her diagnosis was confirmed, we embarked on an emotionally intense journey together—one that is ongoing. We have been through so much. She had a bone transplant, allowing her to elude amputation and keep her affected leg. Four rounds of chemotherapy followed in our attempt to route out and kill the microscopic islands of cancer that are inevitable in this devastating disease. Through it all, she has maintained a quiet elegance and grace that defies description—no complaints, no hard feelings, just trust that her human companions would take care of her.

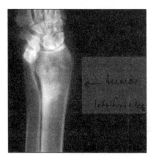

The radiograph of Murphy's bone tumor that started our journey with cancer.

———————— ✣ ————————

In the column I write for *The Denver Post* each Sunday, I shared Murphy's story with my readers. Little did I know that one simple column would lead me to this project, this labor of love. I don't know how much time we have left with Murphy. The odds are against her longterm survival. But we have celebrated our two-year anniversary as of this writing, and every day is a gift.

Within this thin volume, I hope to provide answers to some of the many questions that accompany a diagnosis of cancer in a beloved pet. My goal is to reassure, offer guidance, and show at least a glimpse of what to expect as the journey through cancer management unfolds. If I can assist a single family by dispelling fear and allowing understanding, I will have succeeded.

⌒

chapter one

FACING CANCER: DISPELLING FEAR AND FINDING HOPE

Of all the illnesses we pet owners may face during the life of our pets, none elicits such fear and dread as *cancer*. Cancer is an emotionally charged disease, implying fatality and the impending loss of a beloved pet. Cancer brings lots of unknowns. We don't want to see our animal family members suffer pain, loss of mobility, or loss of dignity. Almost certainly we have all experienced cancer in our lives—either personally or with a family member or friend.

Painful memories may resurface. Each day we may feel helpless or even hopeless. So many emotions surface as we walk this complex path, and so many decisions must be made about diagnosis and treatment. The most important thing to remember about cancer, though, is that it is and remains the single most *curable* chronic disease a pet may face. It has been said that the

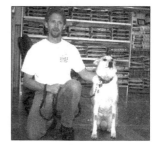

Cancer patient Lady Storm with owner Dan.

———— ✤ ————

❖

MURPHY'S STORY

*Because I am a veterinarian, I am trained to remember always the potential "worst case" scenario. The morning that Murphy, my beautiful black and white Great Dane, limped for the first time my heart sank. One very likely explanation for a limping five-year-old Great Dane is bone cancer. Confirming with a **radiograph** (an X-ray picture) that Murphy had bone cancer in her front leg held double meaning for me. I was just doing my job as her doctor, but I was devastated as her protector and steward. Her diagnosis created a series of life-changing events. Never again will I look at cancer the same way.*

❖
---

color of cancer is black. Yet, despite our initial response to cancer with dread and suspicion, we may replace the blackness of our fear with the light of hope. To do so means taking charge, getting information, creating a plan, and then working through that plan with the pet, the veterinary health care team, and the veterinary cancer specialist.

What will I find in this book to help me?

This book is divided into chapters devoted to individual topics related to pet cancer. The first chapter gives an overview of cancer, its diagnosis, and its treatment and suggests the initial steps to take to help your pet. Chapter two discusses making a complete diagnosis—identifying the type and expected activity of the cancer and uncovering places in the body where the cancer is growing. Chapter three provides a very brief introduction to various treatment options used against cancer. Chapters four, five, and six are devoted to the three most common treatment options used to fight cancer—surgery, chemotherapy, and radiation therapy, respectively. These treatments are often used in combination with one another, depending on what is best for the individual animal. Chapter seven mentions complementary therapies that may supplement traditional treatment. Chapter eight discusses some of the most common emergencies that may arise during cancer therapy. Chapter nine reinforces the importance of nutrition in supporting the pet during cancer treatment. Finally, chapters ten and eleven provide an overview of the decisions we must make as we come to the end of the fight against cancer—providing hospice care and humanely ending the pet's life when control of the cancer is no longer an option.

Immediately following the main text you will find a glossary of many of the terms used in this book. Terms that first appear in italics may be found in the glossary. Following the glossary are resources you may find helpful—suggested additional reading, websites of interest, and a list of veterinary schools in the United States and Canada, including their addresses and telephone numbers.

This book is only an overview—not an exhaustive guide to all the details of cancer diagnosis and treatment. Your primary care veterinarian, the veterinary cancer specialist, and others on the veterinary team are your best resources for answering specific questions that arise about your pet and for helping you create a plan that best fits your needs and those of your pet.

Facing cancer is truly a team effort. You, the caregiver, are at the center of the team—the most important member of the team. Take full advantage of the resources available to you as you travel this journey with your beloved animal companion.

What is cancer?

Cancer is a general term. Cancer is *not* a single disease. The underlying similarity among all cancers is uncontrolled growth of abnormal cells on or within the body. Within most organs or tissues, normal cells grow to replace old cells that have died. Cancer cells, conversely, grow regardless of the need for new cells—they reproduce uncontrollably.

Cancer is the leading cause of death in cats and dogs. It accounts for about half the deaths of pets over 10 years of age. The Morris Animal Foundation Animal Health Survey (www.morrisanimalfoundation.org) revealed that pet owners themselves identify cancer as a leading condition affecting their pets' lives. Cancer is an important and relevant issue for those of us who share our homes with companion animals. There are about 100 different kinds of cancer, and each behaves in a unique fashion once present in the body. Each type of cancer has a specific medical or scientific name. The name of a particular cancer refers to its tissue of origin. For instance, *osteosarcoma* is cancer in the bone. *Squamous cell carcinoma* is a cancer originating in the skin.

What is a tumor?

Groups of abnormal cells form *tumors*. Not all tumors are cancerous. *Benign tumors* are made up of abnormal cells that do not invade or replace surrounding tissue. Benign tumors are usually not dangerous, for they generally do not grow or spread like cancerous tumors. (Another term for a tumor is *mass*.) Benign tumors are most often removed because they grow large enough to cause a problem for the animal, or because they become unsightly. If a benign tumor is diagnosed by noninvasive means like a *needle biopsy* (see the chapter on diagnosis for details), it may simply remain as it is with regular monitoring. When benign tumors grow large or develop an open sore on the surface, they are surgically removed and analyzed. Once removed completely, a benign tumor generally will not recur.

If tumors invade surrounding tissues or destroy and replace normal cells, they are called *malignant tumors*. Sometimes cells from malignant tumors will travel from the original site to other parts of the body via blood vessels or lymphatic channels. They take hold and grow in the new location, making a new tumor. This type of spread is called *metastasis*.

Is cancer contagious?

No. One important exception is feline leukemia virus, which can cause cancer in a cat's lymph nodes and digestive system. In addition, feline leukemia virus causes multiple illnesses that are more typical of infections. Although this disease can spread from cat to cat, the virus cannot spread between cats and dogs, nor can it pass to humans.

Why is cancer so common?

Because our animal companions enjoy the benefits of better nutrition, better preventive health care, advances in veterinary medicine, and closer family relationships, they are living longer. Longer life is a two-edged sword, however. As animals live longer, we see a greater incidence of the diseases that accompany aging. One important example is the increased risk of developing cancer. Dogs develop cancer at a slightly higher rate than humans, whereas cats have a slightly lower incidence rate compared to people. Many factors influence the occurrence of cancer in companion animals. Certain breeds of dogs, like boxers, golden retrievers, and Bernese mountain dogs, are more prone to cancer, pointing to genetic influences in some animals. Pets are exposed to the same environmental toxins (like UV radiation, second-hand smoke, smog, etc.) that humans are. They experience stresses of their own, and we know that stress has an influence on certain cancers in humans.

Could I have prevented my pet's cancer?

Because we do not yet know enough about cancer in animals or people to understand all the reasons why cancer is so common, prevention is elusive. We do know that the incidence of cancer in the mammary glands of dogs is reduced when *ovariohysterectomy* (removal of the uterus and ovaries) is performed prior to the first estrus (heat) cycle. We do know that we can prevent cancer of the testicle in the male dog by neutering. Exposure to second-hand smoke, environmental toxins like 2,4-D, and certain viruses in cats can influence the formation of some cancers. For other types of cancer, however, we simply don't have specific answers yet.

The importance of early detection and treatment cannot be overemphasized. The best prevention of advanced cancer in a cat or dog is a thorough physical examination by its veterinarian—at least twice a year for middle-aged and older pets. Laboratory analysis of blood and urine should be included for it may reveal the presence of disease before the pet looks or acts ill. You should bring any changes in your pet's appetite, activity level, or behavior to the attention of your pet's primary care veterinarian immediately.

How can I tell if my pet has cancer?

Cancer is diagnosed in many different ways, but there are common threads among many different cancers. Sometimes a pet develops an abnormal lump or a bump. Sometimes there is a behavior change—decreased activity, increased sleeping, difficulty getting up and down, decreased appetite, increased thirst, and so on. The Veterinary Cancer Society (www.vetcancersociety.org) has developed a list of the top 10 warning signs for cancer.

1. Abnormal swellings that persist or continue to grow
2. Sores that do not heal
3. Weight loss
4. Loss of appetite
5. Bleeding or discharge from any body opening
6. Offensive odor
7. Difficulty eating or swallowing
8. Hesitation to exercise or loss of stamina
9. Persistent lameness or stiffness
10. Difficulty breathing, urinating, or defecating

No matter what the presenting complaint, any of the signs just listed should prompt a formal examination and diagnostic process. Early diagnosis and treatment are key.

Who will help my pet and my family through the diagnosis and treatment of my pet's cancer?

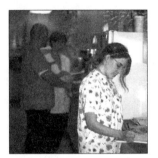

Fighting cancer is a team effort.

———————— ✤ ————————

When facing a diagnosis of cancer in your companion animal, it is critical to remember that the diagnosis and treatment process is a team effort. You will reside at the center of the care-giving circle, for you and your family will provide the day-to-day support your pet needs: giving medication, feeding, bathing, protecting, making decisions. You are the best person to keep in touch with how your animal companion is feeling during cancer treatment. Pets with cancer generally handle their illness and treatment remarkably well. You will be with your pet to help ensure that its quality of life remains high. You will be an important decision maker as treatment progresses. Think of yourself as the captain of your pet's cancer-fighting team.

Your pet's primary care veterinarian and veterinary health care team will serve a pivotal role in coordinating the diagnosis and treatment of your pet's cancer—they know you and your pet and have the best medical perspective of what is normal for your pet. The primary care veterinarian will often perform the workup that provides a complete diagnosis of the cancer (see chapter on diagnosis). This veterinarian will oversee the process, acting as a clearinghouse for information about your pet's progress and outlook. In addition, the primary care veterinarian will provide referrals to appropriate specialists for advanced diagnostics or treatments—the veterinary internist, veterinary radiologist, veterinary surgeon, veterinary cancer specialist, and so on—whoever can best help provide the most positive outcome for your pet.

It is critical, therefore, that your pet's primary care veterinarian instills confidence in you—that you are comfortable working with this individual and his or her staff. Many misconceptions exist about cancer in pets and about the potential outcomes of treatment—even in the minds of some veterinarians. When you are choosing the members of your pet's cancer-fighting team, ask yourself if you prefer a pessimist or an optimist to coordinate your pet's cancer management. It is said that the pessimist not only sees the glass as half-empty but also visualizes a hole in the bottom through which the remaining liquid is leaking. The optimist, conversely, not only sees the glass as half-full but also visualizes the pitcher from which the contents will be replenished.

Most professionals in any field have specific areas of interest and expertise. You can simply ask your veterinarian, "Do you feel comfortable helping me diagnose and treat my pet's cancer?" If the answer is "Yes," then you are probably working with the right individual. If the answer is "No," request assistance in finding a primary care veterinarian who is comfortable, knowledgeable, and optimistic when working with pets with cancer.

In addition, your primary care veterinarian can direct you to individuals and resources within your community to help you and your family with the nonmedical aspects of your pet's illness. These resources include people trained to assist with grief and loss, as well as individuals to help you and your family take care of yourselves while you care for your pet. Remember, you are at the heart of your pet's care-giving team. You must remain sharp, balanced, and healthy.

Parts of the diagnostic plan may involve techniques or equipment unavailable to some practitioners, like magnetic resonance imaging (MRI), computerized tomography (CT) scans, and so on (see chapter on diagnosis for details). Your veterinarian may then refer you to a veterinarian with special training and certification who can complete those procedures. The extended team will also include pathologists who examine tissue under a microscope to provide critical details about your pet's cancer.

Once a complete diagnosis is in place, it is time to formulate a treatment plan. Sometimes all cancer treatment is provided by the primary care veterinarian and his or her health care team, most often in consultation with a veterinary cancer specialist. Sometimes your veterinarian will refer you and your pet directly to a veterinary cancer specialist. Even with a referral to a specialist, your primary care veterinarian will be your most important contact—the one to answer most of your questions and to help deal with any medical emergencies that may arise during treatment.

What else should I think about as I prepare to fight my pet's cancer?
Remember that the veterinary health care team is there to help in any way they can when questions arise or problems occur. You should establish with your team a plan for communication before treatment even begins. What if you have a question about a surgical incision after regular office hours are over? Who will answer your question for you or see your pet at that time? What if your pet seems to have a reaction of some kind to medication that has been given? Who should you call first? Will the primary care veterinarian field most of your questions or will you speak with a veterinary cancer specialist? What if your cat or dog needs to be hospitalized to receive supportive care that can't be provided at home?

Get into the habit of keeping a small notebook and pen with you so that you can jot down questions and concerns as they occur to you. That way you will remember to ask about those things during your next phone call or examination visit. You may also want to write down in your own words the recommendations and comments from the veterinary health care team. Writing things down may make them easier to remember or organize in your mind.

Finally, it is very important that you give all medications according to their directions, in the precise doses, and at the precise times prescribed. It is equally important for you to keep all appointments with your veterinary health care team faithfully. Whether your pet is receiving a chemotherapy treatment, radiation treatment, a laboratory test recheck, or a physical examination, the timing of your pet's visits and treatments is critical for maximum control of the cancer.

MURPHY'S STORY

Once Murphy's diagnosis of bone cancer was confirmed, I set about building her team. I would provide her primary medical care as well as her home care, but there were many other individuals whose help she needed. The veterinary nurses at my practice, as well as the oncology nurses at the Colorado State University Veterinary Teaching Hospital, were invaluable in administering her medications and keeping her comfortable during her treatments. Veterinary oncology surgeons, veterinary medical cancer specialists, veterinary radiologists, and veterinary pathologists at CSU also participated in Murphy's care. In addition, resources provided by the human services team at CSU helped me through the emotional roller coaster I faced early in Murphy's treatment. Without them, we never could have come as far as we have.

$\sim\!\!\circ$

Diagnosing Cancer:
Identifying the Enemy

To provide the best treatment for a cat or dog with cancer, a veterinarian must make a thorough, accurate, and complete diagnosis. No matter what type of cancer a pet has, the approach to identifying the cancer and the extent of the disease must be methodical, involving many steps. What follows is an overview of the diagnostic process.

How is cancer diagnosed?
Step one in diagnosing cancer is a complete and thorough physical examination by your pet's primary care veterinarian, including a rectal temperature. Although cancer itself does not usually cause a fever, occasionally an inflammatory process associated with the cancer may elevate body temperature. (Fever in this case is called a *paraneoplastic event* or *paraneoplastic syndrome—para*, meaning "around," and *neoplastic*, meaning cancer or tumor. This is a symptom or set of symptoms that result from cancer, but which are felt in the body far from the primary tumor site.) The physical examination itself must be systematic in order to uncover any abnormalities in the body either related or unrelated to the cancer.

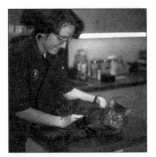

The first step in diagnosing cancer is a thorough physical examination.

— ✤ —

In addition to the physical examination, the preliminary diagnostic plan usually includes a *complete blood count (CBC)*, a *serum biochemical profile*, and a *urinalysis*. The CBC reveals how well the bone marrow is functioning by counting the number of red blood cells, white blood cells, and platelet cells that are moving around in the bloodstream. In addition to counting cell numbers, the analysis identifies which specific types of white blood cells are present and looks at their distribution. Also, the structure of the different types of blood cells reveals important information about their function. The serum biochemical profile includes tests that represent kidney and liver function and that measure blood levels of minerals like calcium, phosphorus, sodium, and so on. Abnormalities in any of these tests help direct further investigation.

For instance, too high a calcium level in the blood (called *hypercalcemia*) can be caused by a cancer that secretes a hormonelike substance that pulls calcium out of the bones and into the circulation. (This is another example of a paraneoplastic syndrome.) Calcium is critical for normal muscle function in the body, including the heart muscle, the skeletal muscles of the limbs, and the smooth muscle of the digestive system. Calcium affects the entire nervous system. Too much calcium can cause cramping in the muscles, disruptions in the heart's rhythm, and kidney damage. If hypercalcemia is detected with the biochemical profile, treatment can be initiated to lower calcium levels back to normal using intravenous fluid therapy.

The urinalysis is an evaluation of the urine, providing information about the urinary tract—how well the kidneys are functioning as they filter waste products out of the blood—as well as revealing abnormal cells that may be present in the urine.

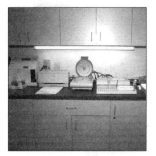

Laboratory tests on blood and urine help make our diagnosis complete.

Following the physical examination and preliminary evaluation of your pet's organ system functions, a more specific diagnostic plan can be formulated. At this point, the veterinarian must identify the tumor and the cell type of origin, define how aggressively the cancer is growing, and uncover where in the body the cancer is present. Also, it must be determined if the cancer cells have spread beyond the primary tumor site, and if organ systems like the liver, kidneys, and bone marrow are affected by the cancer's presence. Only after these facts are gathered can the veterinary team begin to piece together a treatment plan.

How do we identify and define my pet's cancer?

Your primary care veterinarian may first remove a representative sample of the tumor—this is called a *biopsy*. Once a biopsy is collected, it may be analyzed by either the primary care veterinarian or by a specialist to identify the type of tumor, define the tumor's level of malignancy, and help determine what additional diagnostic tests should be done before treatment begins. Defining the level of malignancy of a particular cancer is called *grading* the tumor. Knowledge of a biopsy empowers you and your veterinarian to decide what additional diagnostic tests should be done, what treatment options are available, and what the long-term outlook may be. Biopsies take several forms.

Most tumors lend themselves well to having a small number of cells removed for analysis using a hollow needle and a syringe. This procedure is called a *fine needle aspirate* or a *needle biopsy*. The cells fill the hollow space inside the needle, then are placed on a slide and subjected to special staining that makes them easier to identify. The harvested cells may be analyzed by the primary care veterinarian or a *clinical pathologist*. The clinical pathologist is a veterinary specialist who looks at the small numbers of harvested cells under the microscope, attempting first to identify the cell of origin and then to decide if the cells are cancerous.

A needle biopsy (or fine needle aspirate) should be done when a tumor's location and identification would influence a veterinary surgeon's plan, or when the veterinary team suspects the pet may have cancer present in more than one location. There are certain tumors that are very aggressive, and if present on a leg, for instance, might cause a surgeon to amputate rather than attempt simply to remove the tumor. A needle biopsy is quick, noninvasive, and relatively inexpensive. It provides minimal discomfort for the pet, often yielding accurate results quickly. There are very few disadvantages to a fine needle aspirate, and the procedure is indicated for every tumor that one plans to have removed. The disadvantages of fine needle aspirate (or needle biopsy) include the following:

- The risk of transplanting cancer cells along the track of the needle
- Causing bleeding where the needle is inserted
- Crushing or squashing the cells that are harvested, thereby disrupting their structure and making diagnosis difficult or impossible
- A "negative" result, when the cells that are collected do not provide enough information for the pathologist to make a good evaluation—in this case, the fine needle aspirate may have to be repeated

Another type of biopsy is an *incisional biopsy*. In this case, the veterinarian makes an incision through the skin and into the tumor, removing a section of tissue that ideally incorporates normal tissue around the tumor, a section of transitional tissue at the tumor's border, and a section of the tumor itself. Some tumors, like bone tumors, do not lend themselves well to a conventional scalpel incision, and, in these cases, the veterinarian will use a special instrument that harvests a small core of tissue from the bulk of the tumor. The biopsy is then preserved in a special solution and transported to a veterinary *surgical pathologist* (also called a *histopathologist*) for analysis.

The veterinary surgical pathologist is trained differently than the clinical pathologist who evaluates fine needle aspirates. In addition, some surgical pathologists may be particularly interested in cancer. Ask your primary care veterinarian to be sure your pet's biopsy is evaluated by at least one veterinary surgical pathologist who possesses expertise in evaluating cancer samples. Requesting a second pathologist's opinion in the interest of completeness is absolutely acceptable. Because the sample of tissue in an incisional biopsy is larger than with a needle biopsy, the surgical pathologist is able to assess the tumor more thoroughly than can the clinical pathologist.

Often this type of biopsy provides a definitive diagnosis of the cancer, its cell type of origin, and its potential to spread throughout the body. The zone of transition from normal to abnormal tissue (when it is available) helps the surgical pathologist make a more complete assessment of the tumor. An incisional biopsy is useful when the tumor clearly is too big or invasive to be removed with surgery alone, when the cancer is present in more than one place in the body, or when general anesthesia poses a major risk for the pet.

The goal of an *excisional biopsy* is to remove the entire tumor in one surgical procedure, thus curing the animal of cancer. The tumor itself is removed, including a surrounding zone of visually normal tissue (called the *tumor margin*) to ensure that all the cancer cells are removed. The entire piece of tissue is then submitted to the surgical pathologist for analysis. In this case, the surgical pathologist identifies the tumor type and level of malignancy, plus evaluates the margins of the tumor to ensure that no cancer cells were left behind. The excisional biopsy is well suited to small, superficial masses as well as large, localized, easy-to-remove tumors. The animal must be able to withstand the rigors of anesthesia and surgery. The greatest advantage to an excisional biopsy is the opportunity for cure.

Occasionally, a tumor appears to have been completely removed at the time of surgery, but under the microscope the pathologist either finds cancer cells in the margin of surrounding tissue—called a "dirty" margin because it is contaminated with abnormal cells—or finds that the margins are unacceptably narrow. In this case, the pathology report prompts a second, more aggressive surgery. This is one example of the importance of a complete and thorough microscopic examination of all lumps and bumps that are removed.

Finally, an *endoscopic biopsy* may be the technique of choice. An endoscope has a thin, flexible tube containing fibers that transmit light. These fibers carry a magnified visual image that can then be projected to a video monitor for viewing. The endoscope can be inserted into the body's openings (like the nose or mouth) to visualize and to collect

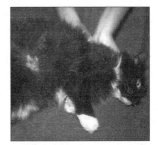

This cat has a tumor in her skin that will be removed and analyzed. This is called an "excisional biopsy."

❖

small samples from abnormal areas on the inside surfaces of the respiratory system, the digestive system, and the lower urinary tract. When inserted into the mouth and passed down the esophagus, the endoscope allows the veterinarian to see tissues and to collect a small biopsy from a mass on the inside surface of the esophagus, the stomach, or the first part of the small intestine. The large intestine and colon can be biopsied by passing the endoscope into the anus. The endoscope can also collect samples from the nasal passage, sinuses, windpipe, and large air passages in the lungs. When passed through the female animal's urethra, the endoscope allows the veterinarian to collect a biopsy from a mass on the inside surface of the urinary bladder. The animal must be strong enough to handle anesthesia for endoscopy, but endoscopic biopsies are far less invasive than opening body cavities surgically to sample tumor cells. Biopsies collected endoscopically are sent to a veterinary surgical pathologist for evaluation.

Besides laboratory tests and biopsies, what other diagnostic tests can I expect for my pet?

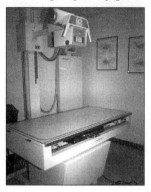

An X-ray machine like this is an important diagnostic tool.

———— ✢ ————

Radiographs (X-ray images) provide a window into the inside of the body. The radiographic image is produced on special film when X rays are passed through a part of the body. The X rays are blocked to varying degrees by the tissues of the body, producing many shades of gray on the radiograph. Denser tissues (like bone) block more X rays and appear white. Soft tissues (like muscle) block fewer X rays and appear gray. Air (within the lungs or outside the borders of the body) blocks no X rays and appears black. Typically, the chest and abdomen are examined radiographically. If any bones in the skeleton seem abnormal on the physical examination, these will also be radiographed. Ideally, a board-certified veterinary radiologist or a veterinary cancer specialist reviews the pet's radiographs. The primary care veterinarian will also benefit from evaluating these radiographs as he or she establishes a diagnosis and develops a treatment plan.

Some facilities use *computerized tomography (CT) scans* as well as *magnetic resonance imaging (MRI)* technology to diagnose cancer, just like for human patients. The CT scan uses computer technology to produce images of cross-sections through the body. Abnormal growths can be visualized as well as measured for their dimensions. MRI technology is also computer assisted. It is particularly well suited for identifying tumors in the soft tissues of the body, like muscles, the lung, or the brain.

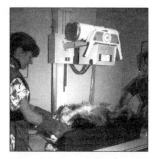

This dog is having radiographs taken of his chest and abdomen as part of his diagnosis.

❖

Once the initial diagnostic tests are complete, do any additional tests have to be done?

After your pet's cancer has been completely diagnosed and treatment has begun, there will be follow-up tests at regular intervals. Your pet's primary care veterinarian will probably coordinate the follow-up process. It is important to monitor your pet for any return or reactivation of its cancer. The type of cancer your pet has and its response to therapy will dictate the tests that should be done. Expect physical examinations, blood and urine tests, radiographs, or a combination of these.

❖

MURPHY'S STORY

Every three months we take radiographs of Murphy's chest looking for any evidence of metastatic recurrence of her bone cancer. If it returns, it will most likely come back in her lungs—that is one of the primary locations for recurrence of bone cancer. We also radiograph her left front leg, examining the site of the bone transplant where her cancer was removed, looking for evidence of local recurrence. We will continue our vigilance for the rest of her life.

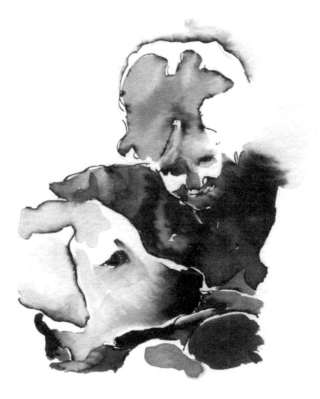

chapter three

⁓

TREATMENT OPTIONS FOR CANCER: AN OVERVIEW

Many treatment options are currently available for pets with cancer. Cancer specialists and scientists create new treatment modalities constantly, both by finding new treatments and by applying existing treatments in novel ways.

One important thing to remember about treating cancer, whether in pets or in people, is that the best approach is usually a multitherapy approach. Such an approach means using two or more treatment options at the same time, versus using only one therapy at a time and using them in sequence. Most often, a combination of treatments is more effective against cancer than one type of treatment alone. The goal is to create the "biggest bang for the buck," maximizing the potential for cure while preventing pain and discomfort and enhancing the quality of the pet's life.

Another critical principle in treating cancer is to maintain a broad perspective. Although it is tempting to zero in on one aspect or another of the disease at hand, too tight a focus may actually impede the fight against the cancer. It is like taking a picture using a telephoto lens versus taking a picture with a wide-angle lens. The telephoto lens gives a detailed view of a very small area. Conversely, the wide-angle lens gives a broad view of a very large area. So it is with treating cancer. The "telephoto view" targets only the tumor we are fighting, allowing the animal patient that survives around the tumor to go out of focus. When battling cancer it is critical to think of the disease within the larger context of the pet's entire being—to keep the "wide-angle view." For cancer treatment to be most effective, the rest of the pet's body and spirit must be sustained and supported. Enhancing the patient's quality of life must remain the highest mission throughout cancer therapy.

What are the most common treatments for cancer in pets?

There are three cancer treatments that are most often used in combination with one another to battle cancer in pets. They are:

- ❖ Surgery
- ❖ Chemotherapy
- ❖ Radiation therapy

What follows is a brief, general overview of these three treatment options. Later chapters provide a more detailed discussion of each.

How is surgery used to treat cancer?

Until the 1950s, surgery was the mainstay of cancer therapy in animals. Most cancer patients at that time were treated with surgery alone.

The intention was to remove all existing cancer cells from the body. Even today, surgery remains the cornerstone of therapy for most cancers in dogs and cats—many times it is curative.

More recent knowledge of cancer and the behavior of different types of tumors reveals that surgery alone is often not enough. Some animals have cancerous tumors too large to be removed safely—the surgery would kill

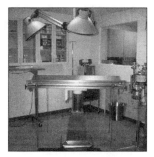

Surgery usually takes place in a room designed specifically for that purpose.

———— ✢ ————

the patient. If an animal has cancer that is either *multifocal* (present in more than one location in the body) or metastatic (cancer cells have moved from the primary tumor to other areas in the body), surgery is often not an effective treatment option.

Even when surgery is not the sole treatment option available, surgery will often play some role in managing the disease. Surgery is an important diagnostic tool for it allows the veterinary team to take a representative section of a tumor (biopsy) for analysis by a pathologist (see chapter on diagnosis). If a large tumor cannot be completely removed from an animal's body, part of the pet's treatment may involve surgically removing as much of the tumor as possible. This procedure is called *debulking*. By decreasing the overall size of the tumor through surgical debulking, other treatments like radiation therapy or chemotherapy may work more effectively. The fewer cancer cells that remain in the body, the better opportunity other treatments have to work.

How does chemotherapy battle cancer?

Chemotherapy involves delivering powerful drugs to the body that kill cancer cells. Chemotherapeutic agents may be delivered by injection into a vein or muscle, injection into a tumor, or orally. The objective is to preferentially kill cancer cells while leaving normal cells alone (or at least providing minimal toxic side effects). Although some humans report adverse side effects from chemotherapy (nausea, vomiting, diarrhea, weakness, hair loss, etc.), dogs and cats seem amazingly tolerant, usually maintaining good to excellent quality of life throughout treatment. Not all cancers are responsive to chemotherapy. Some tumors don't respond at all. Others require chemotherapy to be used in conjunction with other treatments. Chemotherapy tends not to be a cure by itself—rather it provides control over the cancer, for variable periods of time, depending on the type of cancer.

What about radiation therapy?

Radiation therapy uses different types of radiation than what are used to make radiographic images (X-ray pictures, mammograms, etc.). During radiotherapy, radiation is applied to the tumor either via a beam from a machine or, less commonly, via radioactive implants that are placed in and around the mass. When tumors are sensitive to radiation, they sometimes can be cured. At the very least, these tumors will often significantly decrease in size, making surgical removal possible, or allowing chemotherapy to be more effective. Radiotherapy has the potential to be curative for certain tumor sites and types.

Are there any other types of cancer treatment available? For instance, in human medicine "gene therapy" is getting headlines as a new way to fight cancer. What about other options for animals?

There are several additional treatment options for cancer that are not used as commonly as surgery, chemotherapy, or radiation therapy. These treatments currently have limited application, though they may become important options in the future. They include:

❖ Immune modulation therapy/gene therapy
❖ Cryosurgery
❖ Complementary therapy

In *immune modulation therapy*, the goal is to stimulate the body's own immune system in very specific ways to assist in killing cancer cells. Since cancer cells are genetically flawed—mutations of normal cells that then grow out of control—gene therapy to "fix" the mutations present in cancer holds promise, although little data currently exist to document its effectiveness. As newer techniques of genetic engineering are developed, cancer treatment may include genetically "healing" the cancer cells and allowing them to become normal again. At this time, immune modulation and gene therapies are considered supplements to traditional treatments.

Cryosurgery is also effective for certain small tumors in the skin, mouth, eyelid, and anal areas. Cryosurgery involves freezing tumor cells in a very controlled area by the application of liquid nitrogen. One theory is that killing the tumor cells this way stimulates the immune system to "clean up" the area. In certain cases, cryosurgery has the potential to be curative.

Finally, *complementary therapy* involves treatments that are outside the realm of conventional, accepted, proven treatments. These may include acupuncture, herbal remedies, and nutritional therapy. It is important not to replace proven, traditional cancer treatments with unproven ones, but complementary therapies may help support the pet with cancer during conventional treatment.

How will I know what treatments are best for my pet?

Once a complete cancer diagnosis is in place, your primary care veterinarian or the veterinary cancer specialist can suggest treatment options based on their potential effectiveness against the particular cancer the pet is facing. Combination therapy using two or more treatment options is the most common approach to treating cancer today, maximizing the opportunity for a clinical cure. After years of examining the behavior of various tumors in the dog and cat, veterinarians and veterinary cancer specialists can often reliably predict the activity of certain tumor types. Knowing what type of cancer is present and where in the body it resides, the veterinary health care team can anticipate both how the cancer will behave and how it should respond to therapy.

Each treatment plan is formulated for the individual patient, with that animal's quality of life squarely at the heart of the program. Many factors play a part in the decision making:

+ The overall condition of the animal
+ The location of the tumor(s)
+ The pet's potential tolerance of chemotherapeutic agents or the rigors of anesthesia and surgery

- Any previous exposure to chemotherapy
- The projected ability of the pet to adapt to a body-changing surgery (e.g., loss of a limb, loss of an eye, etc.)
- The costs of treatment

It may cost as little as $100 or as much as $6,000 to maintain an animal cancer patient in a cancer-free state for a full year. Costs will vary dramatically depending on the type of cancer and the treatments used. Battling cancer involves a significant investment of emotion, energy, and time, in addition to financial resources.

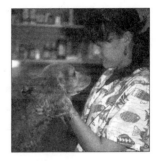

You and the veterinary health care team will work together to formulate the best cancer treatment plan for your pet.

Whatever treatment approach is chosen, cancer therapy is a team process with you, as the caregiver, at the center of the caring circle. Every pet is different. Every household and family situation is different. Ultimately, the animal's quality of life carries the highest priority. Each pet's human family members remain the best qualified (with the input of the veterinary health care team) to make decisions about treatment, supportive care, and the quality of day-to-day life the animal is enjoying. Whether treatment is designed to cure or simply to achieve remission, enhancing the pet's comfort and quality of life are of paramount importance. If treatment causes the animal more harm than good, then that treatment will be modified or abandoned.

How successful is cancer treatment?

Cancer remains the most curable of all chronic diseases. Yet this is the most difficult question of all to answer, for every cancer is different, each having a different prognosis. Early detection and an accurate, complete diagnosis are important keys. Many cancers can be cured. Our current knowledge tells us that over half the dogs and cats with malignant tumors can be rendered completely "cancer-free." Other cancers, although not technically "curable," can be held in check for fairly long periods of time. Even without a cure in sight, most animal cancer patients can maintain a high quality of active life with the help of appropriate treatment. You and your veterinary health care team may choose to focus on remission, however temporary, rather than focusing on cure. Actively and aggressively preventing pain, thus enhancing the quality of life for the pet with cancer, may be the primary concern. No matter what the specific focus, the overall goal is to allow the pet to have the happiest and most comfortable life for the longest possible time.

As our understanding of different types of cancer increases, our ability to do battle with this nemesis of pets will expand as well.

If treated, will my pet's cancer come back?

Even after aggressive treatment, cancer sometimes returns. Cancer that comes back after it has been treated is called a *recurrence*. Recurrence may happen weeks, months, or years after the initial treatment. The period during which cancer remains inactive is called *remission*. The pet with cancer is, by definition, out of remission when cancer returns or is reactivated. The long-term success of treatment depends on many factors, including the type of cancer, the grade of the tumor, where in the body the original cancer was uncovered, as well as the aggressiveness of the initial therapy.

Most often, recurrent cancer originates from cells that have broken away from the primary tumor and have traveled to other parts of the body. Recurring cancer is the same cell type as the original tumor, reestablishing itself in much the same way. For instance, bone cancer that travels to and grows in the lungs is truly bone cancer, not lung cancer. Cancer may recur at or near the site of the original tumor. It may grow in nearby lymph nodes. No matter where it recurs, the goal is to detect reactivated cancer early so that the response may be prompt.

Many cells that break away from the primary tumor are unable to form a new growth. Perhaps the body's immune system, chemotherapy, radiation therapy, innovative treatments (i.e., gene therapy), freezing the primary tumor, or a combination of these are able to stop the traveling cells from developing into cancer.

❖

MURPHY'S STORY

Murphy's cancer treatment combined surgery and chemotherapy. Her surgery removed the bulk of the tumor in her left front leg, replacing the cancerous bone with a transplant from a donor dog. Her chemotherapy included both an implant of slow-release medication at the surgery site as well as medicine injected into a vein. It targeted cancer cells that might have been scattered throughout her body. She tolerated both surgery and chemotherapy exceptionally well.

With each passing year, more information about treating cancer becomes available. Cancer management options are increasingly diverse. More and more pets benefit from creative applications of conventional therapies. Each year more veterinary professionals embrace new understandings of cancer, expanding their abilities to treat these special animal family members. The horizon of hope continues to expand.

chapter four

∼

SURGICAL ONCOLOGY: THE CUT THAT MAY CURE

Surgery has long been the cornerstone of cancer treatment. Surgery is often used to diagnose tumors (see chapter on diagnosis). Surgery is also important in treating many types of cancer—sometimes by itself as well as in combination with other therapies.

What are the advantages of treating cancer with surgery?
The single greatest advantage of treating cancer surgically is the opportunity for an immediate and complete cure with a single surgical procedure. Surgery allows for the most accurate identification of the type of cancer affecting the pet. And for those patients that cannot be cured via surgery alone, surgery may remove a significant number of tumor cells, allowing radiation therapy or chemotherapy to work more effectively.

Sometimes surgery is used to manage side effects of other cancer therapies. Tissue that is damaged during radiation therapy may need to be removed surgically and repaired with a skin graft to help the pet heal more quickly. Surgery is also used to place a feeding tube when a

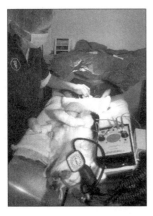

A patient is prepared for abdominal surgery.

———— ✤ ————

pet's cancer or cancer treatment makes eating difficult or impossible.

When a particular cancer cannot be treated with a cure in mind, surgery may enhance the pet's quality of life by reducing the sheer bulk of its tumor or by improving the animal's ability to function. This effect may prolong as well as improve the pet's life. Whenever surgery is considered for a patient that cannot be cured, the potential positive outcome must be weighed against the potential risks.

Should I put my pet through the pain of surgery?

There is a balance to consider before intervening surgically on behalf of an animal with cancer. The benefits must outweigh the risks. The short-term discomfort of surgery must be outweighed by the expectation of a high-quality, pain-free, and disease-free life following the procedure. All members of the cancer-fighting team must be involved in the decision to use surgery. The primary goal of surgery is to remove all (or most) of a tumor while preserving normal (or near-normal) function. The secondary goal is to have a cosmetic outcome. If cancer surgery will prolong comfortable life, then some degree of alteration in appearance or minor loss of function is a worthwhile trade-off.

Postoperative pain can be prevented and managed very effectively with currently available medications. Veterinarians, be they surgeons, veterinary cancer specialists, or primary care providers, are more aware than ever of the negative physical consequences of pain in animal patients. No member of the veterinary health care team wants to see a patient in pain. As a result, the veterinary profession is constantly updating, upgrading, and improving the way pain

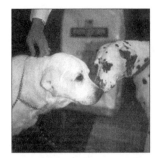

After surgery to remove three different types of cancer, Jessie is going strong at 14 years of age.

———————— ❖ ————————

is prevented in animal patients—especially those with cancer. Consequently, part of your care-giving role will be to monitor your pet's activity and behavior, working with your veterinary health care team to administer medications appropriately to prevent pain.

How will my pet deal with the loss of a body part (e.g., leg, eye, jaw bone)? Will my pet be able to get around on three legs, for instance?
Interestingly enough, humans have much more difficulty dealing with the loss of a body part—their own or someone else's—than animals do. In the case of amputation, as long as the remaining three legs are functional, most cats and dogs can handle the loss of a limb without much adaptation. When part of a jaw must be removed with a tumor, animals are remarkably quick to relearn how to eat, drink, and swallow. When an eye must be sacrificed because of cancer, animals compensate quickly for the loss in depth perception. Cats can learn to climb and jump again after losing an eye. Dogs can fetch again, learning a different way to

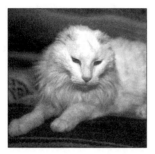

Taffy had surgery to remove skin cancer on his ears. Surgery changed his appearance but saved his life.

———— ✥ ————

watch the ball, toy, or stick that they chase. Pets learn a new body balance for running and jumping after a limb amputation. There are more and more products available for pet owners to use to assist animals who have special physical needs. There are ramps, animal wheelchairs, and supportive straps to help a pet walk with its owner's help.

One important role for the veterinary health care team is to act as a liaison with other families whose pets have had a body-altering cancer surgery (like amputation). Perhaps meeting some of these special pets will help relieve some of the very natural apprehension at making such an important and life-altering decision. By seeing another animal that has adapted to the loss of a limb, eye, or jaw, you may be better able to envision how your own pet may look and act. Hearing the encouragement of other families in a similar predicament may make your load a little lighter.

Will surgery cure my pet's cancer?

Many times surgery will cure cancer, depending on its location, size, and cell type of origin. If a tumor is localized, has little potential to metastasize (spread to other locations), and can be removed with a wide margin of normal healthy tissue, surgery alone is often curative. Even if a tumor is quite large, so long as it is localized and removable with a margin of normal tissue, surgery may be all the treatment required.

Will my pet also need chemotherapy or radiation therapy?

Sometimes surgery alone is not enough to completely cure cancer in a pet. Surgery may be the best treatment to remove or decrease the size of the tumor, preparing the body for follow-up chemotherapy, radiation therapy, or both. With a complete diagnosis and thorough analysis of the tumor, the cancer-fighting team can advise you about recommended follow-up therapy.

What are some of the potential complications of surgery in a cancer patient?

Some of the potential complications from cancer surgery are the same as for any surgery—infection, failure of the sutures closing the incision, and persistent bleeding. Some potential complications, however, are specific for cancer surgery. These include recurrence of the cancer at the incision, unacceptable cosmetic results, and unacceptable loss of normal function. Occasionally, complications can be anticipated and avoided. In other cases, complications from surgery can be anticipated but are unavoidable—such complications may influence your final decision about surgical intervention.

It is important to remember that many, many cats and dogs undergo surgery for cancer each year, and most do not suffer serious setbacks or side effects. If a particular cancer lends itself to surgical intervention, this is an excellent treatment option.

MURPHY'S STORY

Murphy underwent a revolutionary surgical therapy for the bone cancer in her left front leg. The affected section of her leg bone was removed and replaced by bone from a donor dog. The "bone transplant" was matched as closely as possible to the diameter and density of her own bone by matching her radiographs with those of the donor bone. The

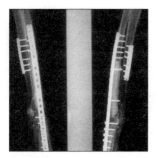

Murphy has two stainless steel plates in her left front leg, one to hold her bone transplant in place and the other to repair her fractured bone.

new bone was secured by a stainless steel plate running the length of her foreleg, fusing her wrist joint. Two weeks after her cancer surgery, she broke the other, healthy bone in her lower left front leg, requiring a second surgery. She is so big that simply walking around loosened her bone plate enough to cause a stress fracture in the other bone.

Following her surgery, Murphy wore a bandage to protect her incision for several weeks, and she took daily doses of antibiotics for several months postoperatively to prevent infection and facilitate healing. We restricted her activity for several weeks (much to her chagrin), but by the four-month mark she was comfortably able to walk a three-mile loop with our other dogs. Four doses of potent chemotherapy followed her surgery, given at three-week intervals. A total cumulative dose of this drug is given when battling bone cancer, after which no more drug is

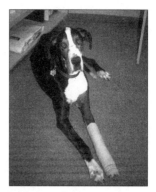

Following her surgery, Murphy wore a bandage to protect her incision.

---❖---

administered. Every three months we look for a return of Murphy's cancer by making radiographs of her chest and left front leg. At the time of this writing, she has passed the two-year mark in her survival. Only 50% of dogs with bone cancer that undergo the same therapy as Murphy live one year.

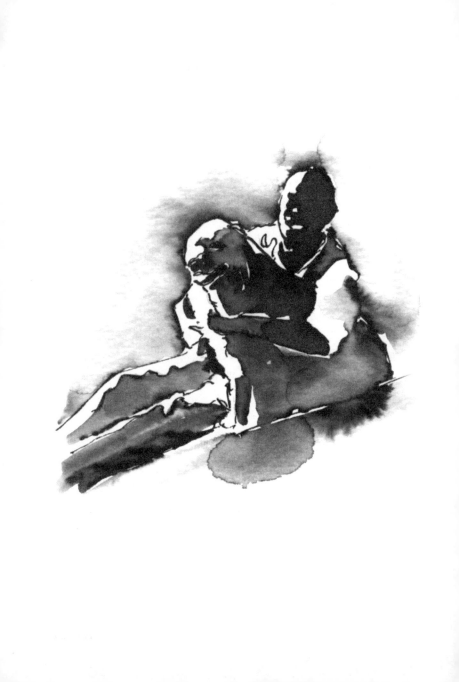

chapter five

~⌒

CHEMOTHERAPY: AN IMPORTANT TREATMENT OPTION

When a pet is ill, only one word is more frightening than "cancer" and that is "chemotherapy." Most of us have had personal experience with someone who has received chemotherapy medication—either a friend or family member, or perhaps even ourselves. Although people can experience a wide range of side effects from chemotherapy, some of them unpleasant, the same is *not* true for cats and dogs with cancer.

Pets with cancer that receive chemotherapy do exceptionally well. Any minimal side effects that may occur can usually be anticipated, prevented, and well controlled. Although we use the same medications to treat cancer in pets that are used to treat cancer in humans, the doses are adjusted for the individual animal's body size. It is important to remember that our own fears about using chemotherapy to fight cancer in pets are generally unfounded and usually reflect misconceptions about what to expect.

What is chemotherapy?

Chemotherapy drugs are very powerful medications that kill cancer cells. Chemotherapy is important in the control of many different types of cancer, enhancing the quality of life as well as increasing survival time. The primary goal in using chemotherapy is to sustain and improve the quality of life for the affected animal. The secondary goal is to stabilize, decrease, or eliminate the animal's cancer. This sometimes stands in contrast to a common attitude in human cancer medicine of "cure at any cost."

Your veterinarian must give the dose of chemotherapy that is most effective to control your pet's particular cancer. He or she will carefully calculate the precise dose to be given. The goal is to get the "biggest bang for the buck," while minimizing side effects. No medication is completely free from all risks for side effects, and chemotherapy is no exception. However, the potential side effects we may encounter are quite variable, and most may be prevented or minimized. Your veterinarian will work with you to ensure that the potential side effects reflect an acceptable risk.

The timing of chemotherapy doses is critical for maximum control of cancer. The dosing interval must be short enough to continue to kill cancer cells without having them develop resistance to the drug, but long enough to allow normal healthy cells to recover. Therefore, it is very important that you keep your pet's appointments with the veterinary health care team faithfully. You and your veterinary team want to be sure to do everything you can to kill as many cancer cells as possible.

How does chemotherapy work?

Chemotherapy works most effectively against rapidly dividing cells—most cancer cells reproduce at a faster rate than normal cells. Chemotherapy drugs selectively target rapidly dividing cancer cells and don't have as powerful an effect on normal cells that divide more slowly. Therefore, the most effective time for chemotherapy is when a tumor is small and the majority of its cells are rapidly dividing. The goal is to use the maximum dose the pet can tolerate in order to kill the greatest number of cancer cells possible per dose.

How do we decide if it is appropriate for my pet to receive chemotherapy?

Step one when treating cancer in any fashion is to get the facts. "Cancer" and "chemotherapy" are words that conjure negative images for many of us because of experiences we may have had with friends, family, or ourselves. It is critical to understand that cats and dogs usually do exceptionally well when treated for cancer—no matter what treatment options we may use. To be the strongest caregiver we can be for our animal companion, we must be armed with knowledge, not myths.

Step two in deciding if chemotherapy is appropriate for a particular dog or cat with cancer is to have a *complete* diagnosis. What type of cancer is present? What is its grade—how aggressively can we expect it to behave? Where in the body is the cancer located? Are there multiple tumors or only one? (See the chapter on diagnosis.) Some types of cancer are well suited for chemotherapy, whereas others are not.

Before deciding to use chemotherapeutic agents, some additional questions must be answered:

- ❖ Is the cancer best addressed by surgery? If it cannot be cured with surgery, would the pet benefit from a surgery that significantly reduces the size of the primary tumor, allowing chemotherapy to act on cancer cells that remain in the body? The smaller the number of remaining cancer cells, the more effective chemotherapy will be.
- ❖ What is the risk that the tumor will spread to other parts of the body or regrow in the original site?
- ❖ Are there effective drugs for battling my pet's particular cancer?

What are the risks to my pet of side effects from chemotherapy?

There are several important applications for chemotherapy. Chemotherapy drugs are used to control cancers that affect the entire body all at once (like lymphoma—cancer of the lymphatic system).

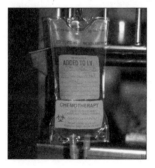

Many chemotherapy drugs are administered intravenously.

❖

Sometimes, when a tumor cannot be removed surgically, chemotherapy offers the best treatment option. If a tumor cannot be removed completely with surgery, chemotherapy is used to fight the remaining cancer cells. Finally, some cancers have a high tendency to spread (metastasize) early in their course (like bone cancer—osteosarcoma—in the dog), so chemotherapy addresses the wandering cancer cells that most likely are present.

Your veterinary health care team will help you decide if chemotherapy is appropriate for your pet. The central focus in cancer treatment is to keep the disease within the larger context of the animal's entire being—not simply to treat a lump or bump. The whole animal must be treated, not just the cancer. There may be particular medical issues (like the presence of kidney disease, abnormal blood counts, etc.) that could influence the choice of chemotherapy drugs or require a dose adjustment. Those adjustments are easily made. Consequently, there are few reasons not to use chemotherapy if it will help to fight cancer.

Remember that cancer is often best treated using more than one therapy, so chemotherapy may be combined with surgery, radiation therapy, or both. In cancer treatment, the strategy is to use the most effective treatments in the safest ways possible.

Is chemotherapy painful for my pet?

No. When administered correctly, chemotherapy is not painful or uncomfortable for the animal cancer patient.

Will my pet lose its hair?

Animals have a different hair growth cycle than humans. Consequently, it is extremely uncommon for them to lose their hair during chemotherapy like we might lose ours. Certain breeds of dogs have hair that requires trimming (e.g., poodles, terriers, cocker spaniels, etc.). These breeds may lose more hair than most dogs during chemotherapy, because they do not have the same shedding patterns as other breeds.

Most cats and dogs that receive chemotherapy are slow to regrow hair in areas that have been shaved for surgery or the injection of medication.

Some animals will grow hair of a different color or texture in these shaved areas once they have had chemotherapy.

Will chemotherapy make my pet sick? What are the potential side effects of chemotherapy?

Most chemotherapy regimens for pets with cancer carry a risk of less than 5% for serious, life-threatening side effects. For the vast majority of animals being treated with chemotherapy for cancer, side effects are mild at most. The potential side effects of chemotherapy reflect the wide variety of drugs that are used to fight cancer, as well as the great variability among animal patients.

Some pets experience an upset stomach (nausea) from certain chemotherapy drugs, resulting in decreased appetite or vomiting. Nausea can usually be prevented and controlled with medication made for that purpose. A pet may develop temporary diarrhea, requiring an adjustment in the meal quantity or feeding schedule.

Some chemotherapy drugs have the potential to suppress the bone marrow, causing decreased numbers of red blood cells, white blood cells, platelets (which help with blood clotting), or a combination of these. The most important of these is a decrease in white blood cells. When white blood cell numbers drop, the animal's resistance to disease is compromised—even the bacteria that live in its own intestines may cause an infection. Blood counts will be monitored carefully during the use of chemotherapy drugs to identify and manage these side effects. If the white blood cell count is too low, your veterinarian may prescribe antibiotics to prevent infection. The dose or timing of chemotherapy may be adjusted if blood cell numbers drop.

There are several very rare potential side effects that can occur from chemotherapy. The best strategy is to review with your veterinary health care team any potential side effects for the particular chemotherapy your pet will receive. Together you will determine if the risk of side effects reflects an acceptable risk. You can then work together to formulate a plan for preventing as many side effects as possible, while preparing a response plan for those effects that are

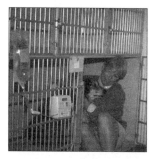

Shadow had a mild episode of vomiting and diarrhea following his chemotherapy. He received IV fluids and a visit from his owner to help him feel better.

❖

unavoidable. Prevention and preparedness are the best insurance against side effects that may occur during chemotherapy.

How are the side effects of chemotherapy treated?
The few side effects from chemotherapy are usually prevented and treated symptomatically. If an upset stomach is anticipated, antinausea medicine is given. If necessary, drugs to protect the digestive tract are given. If a cat or dog becomes slightly dehydrated from not drinking enough, or from vomiting or diarrhea, intravenous fluids are given. This treatment usually results in dramatic improvement and helps the pet feel better quickly. If the white blood cell count drops below a certain level, antibiotics may be given to prevent infection. The dose or timing of chemotherapy may be adjusted if a pet exhibits side

effects. The goal, however, is to anticipate side effects, preventing some and minimizing those that can't be avoided.

How many types of chemotherapy are there?

There are many different types of chemotherapy drugs. There is also much variety in how chemotherapy drugs are used. Some chemotherapy drugs work very well against certain tumors yet are ineffective against others.

The variety of chemotherapy drugs, the many possible combinations of drugs, as well as the multiple administration schedules and cycles make cancer medicine a challenging field. It is no exaggeration to say that new cancer treatments are being discovered, used, and accepted moment to moment. Your veterinarian and his or her health care team will probably coordinate your pet's particular chemotherapy regimen. Your veterinarian may consult with a veterinary cancer specialist to determine which chemotherapy drugs will provide the best treatment for your pet.

How many different drugs will my pet have to take?

Because of the ability of many cancers to become quickly resistant to chemotherapy drugs, often the best strategy is to combine two or more drugs that have different ways of attacking cancer. The ideal scenario is to combine medications that are effective against a particular cancer each on their own, so their additive effect is maximized. With multiple drug regimens, the veterinarian tries to achieve maximum effect against the cancer with minimal side effects to the animal patient.

How long will my pet receive chemotherapy?

No one knows if chemotherapy drugs can truly kill every cancer cell in the body. Depending on the drug and the cancer being treated, some anticancer medications are administered for years after the cancer appears to be gone. One type of cancer for which such a treatment is used is lymphoma—cancer of the lymphatic system. Although it is fairly clear-cut that chemotherapy should be discontinued when a pet's cancer returns or becomes active again, it is not at all clear how long certain medications should be continued after the cancer appears to be eliminated. Some chemotherapy drugs are given for a specific period of time; some are given up to a total cumulative dose.

Will my pet have to be hospitalized during chemotherapy?

Most chemotherapy is administered in the veterinary hospital but requires only a minimal stay for the pet— sometimes a few hours, sometimes a full day. Following chemotherapy, you should plan to clean up body fluids like urine and stool while wearing latex gloves. If your veterinarian feels it is important for your pet to remain

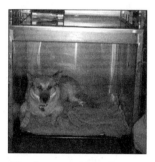

Chuck rests comfortably as he receives IV chemotherapy.

⸙

in the hospital overnight, arrangements can be made to ensure a comfortable stay. Overnight stays are, however, the exception. Sometimes while a pet receives chemotherapy into a vein, a human family member may stay with the animal to help relieve anxiety.

How will we know when to stop the chemotherapy drugs?

Chemotherapy drugs are discontinued in the following situations:

- ❖ When the pet has reached the upper limit of an acceptable total dose for a particular medication
- ❖ When the pet's cancer returns, is reactivated, and seems resistant to that particular drug

If side effects become an important issue, the doses of chemotherapy drugs or the intervals between doses are adjusted and preventive medications dispensed. Usually one is not forced to discontinue treatment because of side effects. These adjustments give you the opportunity to continue fighting the cancer as you focus on making your pet more comfortable.

Throughout a chemotherapy program, it is important to keep appointments faithfully, give supportive medications precisely as directed, and stay in close communication with your veterinary health care team so that any concerns or potential problems may be addressed promptly. You must remember that animals experience very little interruption in their day-to-day lives while undergoing chemotherapy. The few potential side effects that they face can usually be prevented or managed very effectively. For a cancer well suited to chemotherapy treatment, the benefits usually far outweigh the risks.

MURPHY'S STORY

Murphy needed chemotherapy following her "limb spare" surgery. Bone cancer has a bad habit of showing up in the lungs. Her chemotherapeutic agent—cisplatin—had a high potential to damage her kidneys. Part of her treatment included "flushing" her system with intravenous fluids prior to therapy to minimize the drug's potentially negative impact. She tolerated her medication extremely well, though it made her very tired the day of and the day after her therapy. She had no nausea, but she had an intermittent appetite and consequently lost weight after her surgery and during the course of her chemotherapy. She dropped from 148 lbs. to 108 lbs.—always maintaining an excellent attitude, but looking gaunt by the end of her treatment.

Over a six-month period following her final chemotherapy treatment, Murphy regained all the weight she had lost. She now fluctuates between 148 lbs. and 153 lbs. She was a lucky girl to have experienced such minimal side effects.

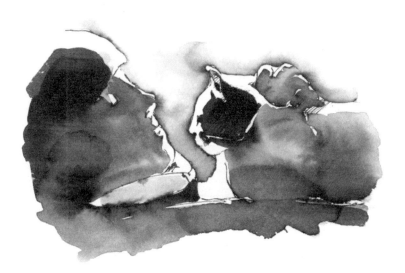

chapter six

RADIATION THERAPY: ANOTHER WAY TO CONTROL OR CURE CANCER

Radiation therapy is very effective in the battle against many different types of cancer. It is used regularly in the management of cancers in humans. Radiation therapy is often combined with surgery or chemotherapy (or both) when a single treatment option does not offer the best potential for maximizing control of the cancer.

What is radiation therapy?

Radiation is a specific type of energy generated by special machines or radioactive substances. A radiation therapist delivers this special energy to a tumor, either in the form of a beam directed at the site of the cancer or via a radioactive implant placed near or into an abnormal growth. Radiation therapy is like surgery in that it is applied specifically to the area of the cancer, rather than to the entire patient. Consequently, any adverse effects of radiation therapy are localized to the treated area. The energy used in radiation therapy is similar to the energy used to make an X-ray picture (radiograph), but it is much more intense. Other names for radiation therapy include *radiotherapy*,

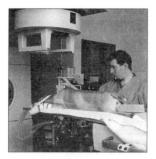

A special unit like this is used to administer radiation therapy. Photo courtesy of Greg Ogilvie, DVM.

———— ✧ ————

cesium or *cobalt therapy, orthovoltage therapy, irradiation,* and *X-ray therapy.*

How does radiation therapy affect cancer cells?

Radiation can directly damage cancer cells, or it can prevent them from growing and dividing. Cancer cells divide faster than normal cells, so they are more sensitive than normal cells to the effects of radiation. In addition, cancer cells cannot repair themselves once they are damaged. The energy of radiation therapy may arrest a tumor's development, or actually cause it to shrink. Normal cells recover faster than cancer cells from the effects of radiation therapy. The radiation therapist strives to balance the intensity of the treatments in a way that maximizes the number of cancer cells killed while minimizing any adverse effects on the surrounding tissue.

Does radiation therapy hurt?

No. When a beam of radiation is applied to a tumor site to kill cancer cells, the animal feels no pain. The energy in the radiation beam does not stimulate pain receptors. Radiation therapy is actually used at times to treat pain and discomfort. In this case, a large, painful tumor may be decreased in size by the application of radiation, providing tremendous relief to the animal patient. Any potential anxiety for the pet is avoided by delivering radiation therapy while the patient is under the influence of a reversible sedative or short-acting anesthesia.

When is radiation therapy used?

There are many tumor types that appear to be sensitive to radiation therapy, alone or in combination with other treatment options. Some examples include certain tumors of the skin, muscle, and nasal passages—all of which occur in both cats and dogs. Radiation therapy works best in a localized area. Sometimes radiation therapy is used to treat a larger area than a surgeon could remove.

Veterinary cancer surgeons sometimes use radiation therapy to shrink a tumor before performing surgery. As a result, surgery may be less traumatic for the pet. Occasionally, a tumor that would otherwise be inoperable is decreased enough in size by radiation to allow the surgeon to proceed. Sometimes a dose of radiation is delivered to the open surgical area prior to closing the incision in order to kill cancer cells that remain at or near the surgical site. This decreases the likelihood of a tumor returning at that location.

Sometimes radiation therapy is used to relieve symptoms associated with a tumor or its spread to other sites, rather than with the intention to achieve a cure. This is called *palliative radiation.* The goal is to enhance the pet's comfort by diminishing the size and activity of the tumor, without necessarily increasing survival time. The timing and number of doses of radiation are different when palliation rather than long-term control of the cancer is the focus.

What are the common side effects of radiation therapy?

During radiation therapy to the head, the tissue that lines the mouth may become irritated and inflamed. This inflammation is called *mucositis.* The development and progression of mucositis is quite variable, and the radiation therapist can help your veterinarian predict its course depending on your particular pet's treatment program. A cat or dog with mucositis develops thick, ropy saliva and bad breath. Since mucositis makes the mouth sore, it is common for the veterinarian to surgically place a soft rubber feeding tube through the side of the neck into the esophagus. Tube feeding allows you to bypass the mouth, delivering adequate nutrition at a time when eating might be difficult for the pet. Any discomfort the animal might feel by eating with a sore mouth is completely eliminated. In addition, the lining of the mouth can heal faster because there is no food to irritate the delicate tissue.

You, as primary caregiver, can do simple things to help your cat or dog with mucositis feel better. Because tube feeding requires a little extra handling of the pet, mealtime becomes a bonding time. Your veterinarian can suggest soothing solutions with which you may flush the mouth to rinse away the thick saliva. This treatment not only cleanses debris from the mouth but also makes swallowing more comfortable. Mucositis usually resolves and the mouth heals within one month of completing radiation therapy.

Sometimes when radiation is delivered to the head, as it is to treat nasal tumors, the eyelids are affected. This can result in irritation around the eyes as well as decreased tear production—called "dry eye." Artificial tears and other eye medications can keep the surface of the eye moist, preventing sores from forming. Decreased tear production may be a lifelong consequence of radiation therapy to the head. Fortunately, most cats and dogs do quite well receiving regular applications of artificial tears—especially if there is a little treat involved!

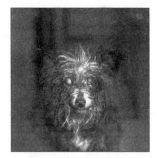

If the anal area is irradiated, the lining of the bowel can become irritated following radiation therapy, causing short-term diarrhea. The pet may need a temporary diet adjustment to control loose stool. The tissue around the anus

Pepper was treated successfully with radiation therapy for a tumor in her nasal passages. Her right eye developed "dry eye," but her cancer was eliminated.

—— ✤ ——

may become irritated. Keeping the area clean and applying prescribed topical treatments will enhance the animal's comfort.

Another effect of radiation therapy involves the skin around a treated area. *Dry* or *moist desquamation* looks like sunburn. The superficial layers of the skin may flake, and the involved areas may be quite itchy for the animal. Desquamation tends to occur at the end of radiation therapy and may take two to four weeks to resolve once therapy is complete. Scratching by the animal makes the condition worse. Your veterinarian can prescribe a soothing solution for you to apply to the affected areas, helping your pet feel better. It is important to use *only* what has been prescribed by your veterinarian. "Booties" on the feet, an Elizabethan collar, or a whole body cover (like a T-shirt) can all be used to prevent a pet from scratching itself.

Even though some side effects from radiation therapy are unavoidable, they vary considerably depending on the area of the body that is irradiated and the dose of radiation that is delivered. Your veterinarian, working with the radiation therapist, can help you to know what to expect for your particular pet. You may find these side effects unsettling and believe them to be uncomfortable for your pet. Remember these effects will resolve in a relatively short time. Remember also, there are simple things—like rinsing a sore mouth, applying soothing solutions and ointments to irritated skin, and so on—you can do at home for your pet to enhance its comfort and quality of life.

Will radiation therapy cure my pet's cancer?
Radiation therapy is most often used in combination with other treatment options. It is the combination that maximizes the potential for cure.

How long does radiation therapy take?
Generally, radiation therapy is given in small doses five days per week for three to six weeks, but this schedule can vary greatly depending on the type of cancer, the pet's response to therapy, and the long-term goal. Palliative radiation, for instance, may only be given once weekly for three to four weeks, or even daily for one to five treatments. Although the actual time of exposure to the radiation beam during each treatment is quite short, there is a fair amount of preparation time. Sedation or anesthesia is required for each radiation treatment to ensure the animal doesn't move.

---- ✦ ----

MURPHY'S STORY

Murphy's treatment regimen for bone cancer did not include radiation therapy. Some radiation oncologists, however, are currently working with veterinary surgeons to explore the option of using radiation therapy to kill bone cancer cells during surgery, maintaining the dog's own bone in its leg rather than replacing it with a bone transplant.

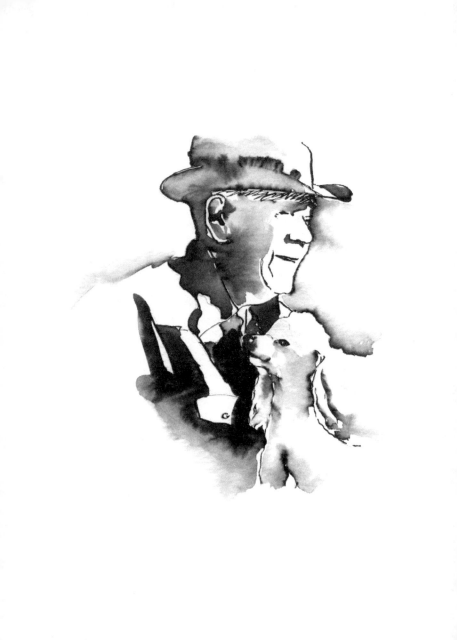

chapter seven

Complementary Therapies: Expanding the Battle Against Cancer

The term "complementary therapies" implies treatments that are outside the realm of conventional, accepted, proven treatments. One study showed that one-third of all Americans routinely pursue complementary therapies for their own health care—particularly as a supplement to traditional health care. A similar trend is occurring in veterinary medicine. Animal cancer patients sometimes face limited treatment options. Complementary therapies that support the animal during traditional cancer treatment are appealing. These therapies include acupuncture, treatments to modify the immune system to fight cancer cells, and gene therapies that attempt to block a cancer's ability to spread in the body. Unfortunately, few traditional data exist about the efficacy of many nontraditional medical modalities. Many treatments that have been used for generations in other cultures simply have never been subjected to the type of clinical study common in our Western view of things.

Sometimes untried and untested methods for fighting cancer are held forth as the "next wave" of therapies. We see this happen in cases of human cancer. Unproven therapies should not replace the pursuit of traditional, proven treatments. It is important not to allow false hopes and empty promises to lure us into subjecting our animal companions to potentially unsafe treatments, especially if we are reaching the end of the fight when every moment of togetherness is vitally important.

What are some examples of complementary medical treatments?

Acupuncture is an ancient form of medicine that originated in Asian culture more than 2,000 years ago. It addresses the body from a very different perspective than our Western medical mind-set. The focus is on

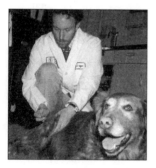

Acupuncture involves stimulating specific points on the body by a variety of means. This dog is having acupuncture applied with needles. Photo courtesy of Greg Ogilvie, DVM.

reestablishing balance in the body by modifying the way energy flows through the body along parallel channels called *meridians*. Acupuncture involves stimulating specific points on the body using needles, heat, electromagnetic energy, friction, or a combination thereof. Acupuncture is applied more and more often in veterinary medicine. Acupuncture is one of the most commonly used and studied complementary medical techniques.

Chiropractic medicine is a treatment modality that stresses the relationship between structure (primarily of the spine) and function (primarily of the nervous system). Manipulation of the spine and limbs realigns body structures and allows healing to occur. Data support the efficacy of chiropractic in human medicine, but few data are available about chiropractic care of the cancer patient. For the animal cancer patient, the focus of chiropractic care is to reduce pain and improve function and mobility.

Massage therapy is another complementary medical treatment that involves manipulation of body tissues, with a focus on the muscles, circulation, and the nervous system. Although few data are available demonstrating the efficacy of massage in animals, massage has been shown to relieve chronic and acute pain, chronic and acute inflammation, nausea, tissue swelling, and anxiety in humans. Massage also releases endorphins in human patients—naturally produced chemicals that can block pain and contribute to an increased sense of well-being. This effect of massage may also occur in animals. For the animal cancer patient, massage is most important in relieving pain and maintaining function.

Homeopathic medicine involves the use of remedies made from naturally occurring substances—primarily plants, animals, and minerals. The remedies are usually diluted to extremely low concentrations such that only the energy or essence of the substance being diluted remains. The theory is that the electromagnetic energy of the molecules in the remedies interacts with the body, providing a healing effect. Homeopathy may support a cancer patient by relieving symptoms of the cancer. Few data support the use of homeopathic remedies to treat or prevent cancer in humans. Among veterinary patients, data involving homeopathic remedies are limited.

Pharmacological and biological treatments involve drugs and vaccines that are not yet accepted by the traditional medical establishment. One example is *cartilage products*—these are derived from the cartilage of sharks and cattle. Unproven reports from other countries imply that shark cartilage is effective in treating cancer in people. Well-controlled, scientific studies have yet to demonstrate this product's effectiveness in humans. One report in the veterinary literature did not support its effectiveness in animal cancer patients. Another example of a biological treatment is called *immunoaugmentive therapy.* This is an experimental cancer treatment that involves injecting blood products daily into the animal cancer patient. Early data suggest that dogs with bone cancer may benefit from this type of treatment. The immune system may be stimulated by factors in the injected materials.

Herbal and botanical medicines are used by about 4 billion people worldwide, though acceptance differs widely. Studies in Europe have generated the best data about the efficacy of these remedies. Some of the herbal agents used in China have been adapted for use in humans for Western-style cancer treatment.

Nutritional therapy presumes that specific nutrients can treat and support individuals with cancer—both human and animal. Some theories advocate supplementation with specific nutrients—like n-3 fatty acids or vitamin C—to treat or prevent cancer. Other theories recommend revising the entire diet to reflect a specific emphasis—like a vegetarian diet. Lifestyle diets, like those found in the Mediterranean countries and Asia, have been studied at length and have been found to decrease the risk of heart disease and cancer in humans. Subsequent research in veterinary medicine has lead to formulation of specialty diets that support animal cancer patients and inhibit the spread of cancer in the body (see chapter on cancer and nutrition).

How can acupuncture help an animal cancer patient?

Acupuncture may not be able to treat a pet's cancer directly—that is, stop a tumor from growing—but it may be very effective in helping to control

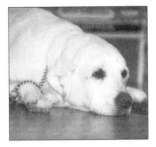

Acupuncture helped Jessie to move around more easily and comfortably.

❖

pain associated with cancer in pets. Throughout the veterinary community, it is becoming easier to find certified veterinary acupuncturists. The primary care veterinarian or veterinary oncologist can make a referral to a competent veterinary acupuncturist to assist in the management of cancer symptoms.

In addition to managing pain, acupuncture may help an animal cancer patient feel better in general and may boost the immune system to better battle the disease. Acupuncture can also help to decrease nausea and increase appetite in pets with cancer. Adequate nutritional support is critical in these animals, and any way we can increase appetite and calorie intake benefits the pet in its fight against cancer. Overall, acupuncture may be a useful tool for enhancing the quality of life for animal cancer patients. Acupuncture remains one of the most common complementary medical modalities used in animal cancer patients.

Are there vitamins or herbs that may benefit my pet?

Although it is well established that omega-3 fatty acids will help prevent cancer cachexia (see chapter on cancer and nutrition), other vitamins, minerals, and herbs have not yet been proven by traditional Western scientific methods to benefit pets with cancer.

That said, your primary care veterinarian can provide a referral to a veterinarian whose practice focuses on complementary medical methods should you choose to pursue any and all appropriate treatments that might help your pet better face its disease. There are specific complementary tools available to help pets feel better during the course of cancer treatment.

⚘

Cancer and Nutrition: Feed the Patient, Starve the Tumor

Cancer has far-reaching effects throughout the body, including the disruption of metabolic pathways and functions. This disruption causes metabolic chaos, robbing the pet of the ability to extract adequate useful nutrition from the food it eats. Research shows that these metabolic alterations persist, even when the animal's body has been cleared of the cancer. One important goal in managing the animal cancer patient is to support the pet while making it more difficult for the cancer to survive—in essence, we want to "feed the patient, starve the tumor."

Simply having cancer and undergoing treatment is a draining experience. Many animals undergoing cancer therapies have periods of inappetence, nausea, or difficulty chewing or swallowing. These are all animals that require special attention to their nutritional needs. They may need special feeding methods or medicine to make eating easier. Not only must we pay close attention to the type of food that is fed, we must be certain to get those calories into the body in the first place. It is imperative that pets with cancer eat *something* rather than nothing, but if they *will* eat, there is now solid scientific guidance about *what* to feed them.

When battling cancer, we are not just fighting a tumor—we are not simply targeting a "lump." It is critical when considering cancer to keep the disease within the larger context of the animal's entire being. By doing so, the focus is on the whole body, not just the small part of the body that is affected by cancer. For cancer treatment to be effective, the remaining healthy parts of the body have to be supported and remain functional.

I have known pets with cancer. Some became very thin despite eating well. What happened?

The nutrients that are absorbed from the digestive tract usually provide fuel for the body. Cancer interrupts the metabolic functions, short-circuiting the body's efforts to energize itself. The tumor preferentially takes over the energy-generating pathways. The body gets the "leftover" energy, which means operating at a loss, while the cancer thrives. The result is a very specific state of accelerated starvation called *cancer cachexia*.

Cancer cachexia actually occurs before weight loss begins, but in its more advanced stages, cancer cachexia has a characteristic appearance. The affected pets lose fat and then begin to lose muscle mass. Their bodies become "shells." Even if they continue to eat well, unless they are eating a pet diet designed to support the cancer patient, the wasting continues inexorably. The result is decreased quality of life, shortened survival time, and decreased response to treatment compared to animals that are not dealing with cachexia.

Since my pet likes its regular food, why can't I just feed that? Why is its regular food a problem now that my pet has cancer?

There are three basic sources of energy found in food—carbohydrates, proteins, and fats. These three energy sources are absorbed from the food the pet consumes and are used as building blocks within the body. Many commercial pet foods are fairly high in carbohydrate and contain moderate levels of protein and fat. Unfortunately, cancer wreaks its greatest havoc within carbohydrate metabolic pathways, monopolizing the energy produced there for itself and leaving the body with a net energy loss. It is this net loss that accounts for the weight loss of cancer cachexia—the body is forced to use its own tissues as a source for the energy simply to survive. As a result, pet diets high in carbohydrate (simple sugars)—that is, many commercially available pet foods—should be avoided by animals with cancer. Since both the body and the tumor require protein, there is no advantage in simply increasing the amount of protein fed. In addition, fat metabolism is also unbalanced, and fat loss is the majority of the weight loss experienced by cancer patients. Regular, commercially available pet foods simply are not "built" to help the body withstand the imbalances that occur with cancer.

Can't I just feed more food (more calories) to prevent weight loss?

Unfortunately, the issues involved in the nutritional support of animal cancer patients are far more complex than simply the number of calories the pet consumes. The types of calories (carbohydrate, fat, and protein) and the blend among them are at the heart of maintaining adequate nutrition and preventing weight loss.

How can I best feed my pet now that it has cancer?

One very important breakthrough in the field of cancer nutrition uncovered the importance of fat calories in a diet when total calorie content and protein content were held constant. The research so far has concentrated on dogs with cancer, so statistics and nutritional percentages quoted refer specifically to dogs. Data on cats will be forthcoming.

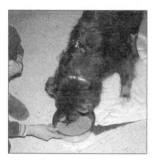

Hill's® Prescription Diet® Canine n/d® is the first commercially prepared specialty food for dogs with cancer. Although it is important that animal cancer patients eat well each day, it is best if they eat a diet designed to feed the patient and starve the tumor. Photo courtesy of Greg Ogilvie, DVM.

❖

A *canine* cancer patient supported with a diet containing 35–50% of nonprotein calories from fat tends to remain in a positive rather than negative energy balance and may actually gain weight. This means a protein calorie density of 25–40%, with carbohydrate levels of no more than 10–30% (compared to carbohydrate calorie density in the 50–60% range for the average canine maintenance diet). One commercially prepared specialty food, manufactured by Hill's® Pet Nutrition—Prescription Diet® Canine n/d® —is now available for dogs with cancer and addresses these nutritional details.

The veterinary cancer specialist, working with the primary care veterinarian, can assist with modifying an existing cat food to accommodate the metabolic changes present in the feline cancer patient. There is not as yet a commercially available feline ration that supports the cat nutritionally in the face of cancer.

One additional breakthrough for the animal cancer patient is the recognition that specific fatty acids—known as "n-3" or "omega-3" fatty acids—assist the body in battling cancer (the research was done in dogs, but the results may also prove true for cats). This translates to increased remission times, decreased spread of the cancer to other locations in the body, and in general to improved quality of life. These fatty acids (think of them like vitamin "F") come from fish.

Once my pet's cancer is in remission, can I start feeding his regular food again?
Unfortunately, the metabolic imbalances that occur when cancer invades the body appear to persist for months or maybe years. Even when cancer is effectively cured, the body's metabolic functions may not return to normal. Consequently, the nutritional support put into place during cancer treatment should remain in place once the treatment is complete. If a dog with cancer is eating Hill's® Prescription Diet® Canine n/d®, that food is probably the long-term diet of choice. For a cat, any dietary modifications made with the input of the veterinary cancer specialist should remain in place for life. As more information becomes available, dietary guidelines for the veterinary cancer patient will continue to evolve.

Can my pet's diet prevent cancer?

Although we now know we can make good choices for nutritional support of animals once they have cancer present in the body, so far there is no indication that any particular feeding regimen will actually prevent cancer. There may come a time when we will have more understanding of specific ways in which cancer in pets can be avoided.

What if my pet stops eating during cancer treatment?

Caloric support is critical during the course of cancer treatment. The patient's body must be nourished to stay strong. There are many reasons why a pet may stop eating when it has cancer and is undergoing therapy.

The tissue that lines the digestive system is very sensitive to radiation. During radiation therapy, the mouth and throat may become temporarily blistered and sore, discouraging the animal from eating and drinking. The lining of the lower digestive tract may also sustain temporary damage during radiation treatment, resulting in diarrhea. The diarrhea may in turn cause nausea, which also decreases appetite. Any surgery performed on an animal cancer patient has the potential to cause that pet to lose interest in food as it is recovering from the operation. Surgery to remove a cancer in or near the mouth may involve removing a part of the upper or lower jaw. While the pet adapts to using its "new" mouth, it must be supported with appropriate nutrition.

It is under circumstances like these, however, that pets most need optimal nutritional support. The veterinary health care team, as well as the oncology team, must be alerted so that they can develop a strategy for a pet with cancer that is either unable to eat or uninterested in eating.

It sounds as though nutrition is fairly important in the overall management of my pet's cancer. Is that true?

Remember that treating a pet with cancer means treating and supporting the entire patient, not just a disease entity we call "cancer." One way to support the bodies of animal cancer patients is to use treatment options that only target cancer cells. Chemotherapy kills cancer cells but allows healthy normal cells to continue functioning. Radiation therapy kills cancer cells or sensitizes those cancer cells to absorb higher levels of lethal chemotherapeutic agents. Other treatment strategies employ the same selective targeting of malignant cells, allowing normal cells the opportunity to maintain.

Because of the shifts that occur in an animal's metabolic processes when cancer is present, "normal" tissue may cease to function in a normal fashion. Overall, the body loses energy, despite what should be an adequate intake of calories. This "energy vampire" character of cancer must be addressed or treatments that might otherwise make a positive difference fail in the face of a body that "fades away." To have the greatest positive impact on the "animal that surrounds the cancer," it is critical to continue to "feed the body and starve the tumor" by focusing on nutrition for the remainder of the animal's life.

❖

MURPHY'S STORY

Murphy has had a dramatic response to the introduction of Hill's®
Prescription Diet® Canine n/d® into her life. We call it her "cancer
diet." She has regained a slick, shining, soft hair coat. More important,
though, she has regained the weight she lost during her chemotherapy
program. She has recaptured her precancer stamina and energy level.
She is thriving, for we are feeding her and not her cancer.

❖

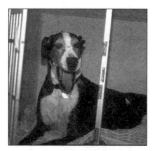

Murphy looks forward each
day to her Hill's® Prescription
Diet® Canine n/d® . She is
thriving and feels terrific!

—— ❖ ——

Nutritional management for the animal
cancer patient does not only mean
focusing on the food a pet eats. It also
means paying attention to getting the
appropriate number and balance of
calories *into* the pet's body. If a particular surgery has changed the way an
animal's mouth works, requiring the
pet to learn a new way of picking up
and chewing food, the animal may not
be able to eat enough during the
learning period to adequately support
itself. Sometimes cancer surgery of the
upper or lower jaw or of the tissues inside the mouth requires a certain
amount of time to heal. The tissue may be tender enough during the

healing time to make normal eating impossible. Radiation therapy can wreak havoc on the lining tissue of the mouth and throat. These rapidly dividing cells may be as affected by the radiation as are the cancer cells being targeted. The resulting inflammation of the oral tissues—called mucositis because it involves irritation of mucous membranes—causes excessive drooling and difficulty swallowing and can make a pet miserable if it attempts to eat.

In these latter examples, the animal cancer patient must have alternatives to the ways in which it would normally eat. This means bypassing the mouth, and sometimes means bypassing the entire upper digestive system.

How can I "bypass" the mouth and throat unless my pet is going to be fed intravenously?

The best way to support any animal that is dealing with devastating disease is by ensuring adequate nutrition. Even in human medicine, the conventional wisdom is to use the digestive system if it is available for us to use. Nutrients are best presented to the body and best absorbed via the digestive system. Unfortunately, intravenous feeding (called *total parenteral nutrition* or *TPN*) is not as effective or as well balanced for animal patients as it is for human patients. It is not the best choice for most animal cancer patients.

One excellent tool for bypassing the structures of the mouth and throat is the *nasogastric (N-G) tube.* Just as the name implies, this is a small-diameter, soft, pliable rubber tube that passes through one of the nostrils, through the nasal passages, and down to the very end of the esophagus or into the stomach. The tube is usually secured along the outside of

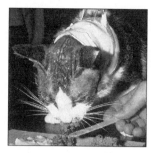

An esophagostomy tube is an excellent way to bypass the mouth yet maintain adequate calorie consumption. Photo courtesy of Greg Ogilvie, DVM.

❖

the body by sutures. In addition, most pets that need an N-G tube must wear an Elizabethan collar around their necks. This apparatus resembles a lampshade. It is worn around the neck and prevents the pet from using its front or hind feet to dislodge the N-G tube. A nasogastric tube must be extremely small to rest comfortably in the nasal passages of pets, making this a difficult feeding method for cats. The smaller the tube diameter, the tougher it is to find a feeding product with the appropriate consistency and texture. Animals tend to object a bit more when a tube is positioned through a nostril, for the tube touches the exquisitely sensitive tissues of the face and muzzle.

Another effective tool for bypassing the mouth and throat of cancer patients during healing is the *esophagostomy tube*. This soft rubber tube is placed during an ultrashort general anesthesia procedure—it requires no special equipment, may be placed in about five minutes, and is almost always well tolerated by the animal. The tube enters the left side of the neck below the angle of the jaw, passing into the esophagus. The delivery end of the tube is positioned at the end of the esophagus without entering the stomach so no stomach juices can irritate the esophagus. The feeding end of the tube, which is outside the body, is secured by sutures to the skin of the neck in several spots, after which the neck is covered in a light wrap. The pet is then fed a gruel consistency food that is passed through the tube with a syringe. Esophagostomy tubes can remain in place for a long time comfortably, and they actually interfere very little with the animal's lifestyle. This feeding technique is particularly effective and well tolerated in cats. Some cancer patients are fed comfortably through an esophagostomy tube for years.

Finally, some patients are best served by special tubes that allow delivery of nutrients directly into the stomach—*gastrostomy tubes (G-tubes)*—or into the small intestine—*jejunostomy tubes (J-tubes)*. The veterinary health care team will determine which nutritional intervention technique (if one is needed) is best for a particular pet.

The most important point is that any cat or dog facing cancer has little room for nutritional compromise—both from a mechanical and a metabolic standpoint. The data are clear that nutritional adjustments must be made in the pet's diet to support the body without inadvertently supporting the cancer. Any potential obstacles to the pet's ingestion of enough of the "right" foods must be anticipated and overcome. We must prevent the negative energy balance that causes insidious and irreversible weight loss.

Paying attention to the nutritional management of a companion animal with cancer brings that pet and its human companions closer than ever. In our society, "food" often equals "love." When we care about someone, we invite him or her into our home for a meal together. For the cat or dog with cancer, good nutrition provides a critical link to life, wellness, and healing. With each meal we help our animal family member to fight the ravages of disease.

Nutritional therapy brings the animal patient and care-giving human family members closer than ever, facilitating the healing power of love and support. As we attend to the details of feeding pets with cancer, we tend to "spoil" them even more than usual. Meal times become important bonding times. The extra petting, hand feeding, and verbal encouragement enhances the mind-body response. Research in human cancer patients has shown that the mind-body connection influences improvements like decreased hospitalization, enhanced immune-system function, and increased survival time. It makes perfect sense that we may have the same positive results when we work to "feed the patient, starve the tumor."

chapter nine

⁓

HOSPICE CARE FOR PETS: WHEN CANCER THERAPY NO LONGER HELPS

Cancer remains the most curable chronic disease facing cats and dogs. Unfortunately, cancer therapy does not always result in a complete cure. In many cases, treatment provides a period of remission, followed by a return of the cancer. There may come a time when the *quality* of your pet's life is more important than the *quantity*. At that point in an animal companion's life, the focus shifts from "cure at all cost" to "aggressive comfort treatment"—a phrase coined by Dr. Eric Clough, a pioneer in the area of veterinary hospice care. Compassionate comfort care as we approach the end of a pet's life allows us to provide both quality of life and quality of death.

The truth is that once cancer therapy options are exhausted or are no longer effective, there is still much to be done to manage pain and provide comfort for the pet as the end of life draws near. This is what *hospice care* is all about.

What exactly is hospice care?

Hospice care is compassionate care that is administered to the animal patient prior to euthanasia, but after control of the cancer becomes ineffective. Hospice is a philosophy, not a physical place. Hospice care focuses on living with dignity in the face of an illness. Hospice provides kind, safe, pain-free, end-of-life care at home for the animal companion. It is especially appropriate for the pet whose cancer has returned or is reactivated.

Hospice care had its beginnings in England in the 1960s in human health care as an alternative to the cold, impersonal death so common in a hospital setting. The goal was to provide the terminally ill patient and his or her family with the opportunity to depart this world in the comfortable, familiar, intimate setting of home.

Applying the principles of hospice care to terminally ill animals seems a natural choice. The animal's human companions benefit from the opportunity to do special things for the pet—special treats and other gifts of time and energy. It gives us—especially children in the family— time to come to grips with the pet's progressive, terminal illness. Hospice care gives a family time to say good-bye. The pet benefits during hospice care from the many true contributions to its quality of life—extra physical affection, favorite food treats, and extra one-on-one time with family members.

When considering hospice care, each animal patient is assessed individually and a plan of care developed. Aggressive treatment with the intention of cure must be contrasted with palliative care that is designed to comfort. The veterinary health care team can help during this difficult decision. If aggressive cancer therapy will not change the outcome, will in and of itself cause harm, or will compromise the quality of a pet's life, hospice may be the best choice. Hospice is appropriate when the animal's illness is terminal and when quality of life is the primary focus. If the diagnosis is complete yet treatment of the cancer itself is ineffective, and visits to the veterinarian come too often, perhaps hospice is the answer. When a

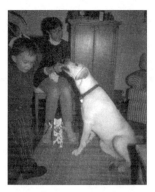

Hospice care supports the precious relationships we have with our pets.

——————— ❖ ———————

cat or dog cannot recover from its cancer, time in the hospital takes away precious "together-time" from the pet and its family. Hospice returns this valuable time.

Will my pet be in pain if I decide to discontinue cancer therapy (like chemotherapy or radiation therapy)?

Every pet owner's greatest nightmare is that a pet will suffer pain or fear during an illness—terminal or otherwise. Pain is defined as an unpleasant sensory and emotional experience associated with actual or potential tissue damage, or described in terms of such damage. Cancer varies greatly in the level of pain it causes. Discontinuing cancer therapy does not necessarily mean a pet will be in pain. The veterinary health care team will provide important information regarding the potential for pain of particular types of cancer. For the animal with cancer whose end is approaching, pain management takes a higher and higher priority.

The best way to manage pain is to *prevent* it. Referred to as *preemptive pain management*, this strategy anticipates discomfort and medicates ahead of that time. It is more difficult to relieve pain once it is present. The pet may become agitated, upset, vocal. Higher doses of medication are then required to control the symptoms, which increases the risk of negative side effects of the pain medication. By medicating "by the clock" instead of by indications that pain is present, you can ward off painful experiences for the animal patient. The veterinary team will prescribe pain medication and doses, as well as a dosing schedule based on how long the drug is active in the body. In addition, there will be quick-acting drugs available for times when the regularly scheduled medication isn't quite enough. Pain medications vary in their strength and length of activity. The veterinary team will begin with less potent medications and work up to the very powerful drugs as the need arises.

If my veterinary health care team and I decide to provide hospice care for my pet at home, does that guarantee that my pet will die on its own? Will I still be faced with making a decision for euthanasia?

Hospice care is not a substitute for euthanasia. Although some animals will die on their own at home during hospice care, the majority must rely on human family members to understand when their quality of life is unacceptable. That means making the difficult choice for euthanasia when the time comes.

I don't want my pet to suffer with its cancer. How can hospice care prevent that from happening?

The focus of hospice care is intimate, nurturing, end-of-life care at home. Home care puts human family members in the unique position of "tuning in" to day-to-day nuances in the animal's attitude, appetite, ability to get around, etc. Hospice empowers the family to take an active role in relieving discomfort and suffering in the cat or dog with cancer. The increased daily attention to details heightens everyone's awareness of how the animal is doing. Through the use of preemptive pain management, nutritional support, physical affection, and increased contact time with human family members, hospice care provides for pets with cancer in a way that helps to prevent pain, isolation, fear, and suffering.

Pain management carries the highest priority during hospice care. Other symptoms of cancer cannot be effectively addressed until pain is controlled. Addiction to pain medication in pets is not a concern because of the circumstances of pain control in the animal cancer patient. The need to prevent discomfort far outweighs any issues around an animal's dependence on medication. Also, psychological issues weigh heavily in human addiction to pain medications. Fortunately, animals don't face these same mental and emotional issues.

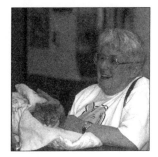

One key to hospice care is keeping visits to the veterinary hospital to a minimum.

❖

Your veterinary health care team is as committed as you are to ensuring that your pet does not suffer pain or discomfort during cancer treatment or hospice care. Take advantage of their knowledge by asking any and all questions that occur to you as you work with them to formulate your pet's treatment plan.

If I am providing hospice care at home for my pet with cancer, how will I administer medications—particularly if my pet is reluctant to eat?

Fortunately, modern medicine has provided many strategies for delivering medication. The oral route is usually the easiest, so it is used most often. Medication can then be hidden in a bit of food and delivered in a meal. For medications that cannot be given orally, injection may be the delivery method of choice. Some medicine is administered rectally, via a tablet that is designed to dissolve in the rectum, or via a soft suppository.

How will I know that it is time for my pet to die?

The most difficult decision any of us face who share life with an animal is the decision to end that animal's life. Even in the face of a terminal disease, the actual decision remains an agonizing one. One strategy for anticipating euthanasia is to establish a family "bottom line" for the pet with contributions from all human family members. This means defining for the family what "quality of life" means. The veterinary health care team can provide invaluable input.

There are many criteria to think about when considering quality of life issues—many questions that must be answered:

- Is the pet able to groom itself and keep itself clean? This is an especially important issue for cats.
- Is the animal able to eat and drink on its own? Sometimes an animal with cancer requires a feeding tube temporarily while healing from a surgical procedure, or during the acute effects of radiation therapy. This is not the same situation as the animal that no longer has any interest in food. In this latter case, a feeding tube is a heroic measure that may artificially prolong a questionably comfortable life.
- Does the pet recognize its surroundings? Can it find its way around the house? What about moving around the yard (if applicable)? Is the animal able to move about at will?
- Is the pet able to control urine and stool output?
- If laid on its side, can the animal "right" itself—that is, get itself into an upright position?
- Does the pet recognize and greet human family members? Some dogs, for instance, seem to "smile" when they greet their humans. Many cats vocalize as though saying "Hello."

These assessments are examples of parameters that are used to evaluate the animal's functional status. In addition, the animal's clinical signs are used as a benchmark. When the following symptoms worsen or are difficult to control, the time may be approaching for euthanasia.

- Fluid retention and bloating
- Dehydration
- Weight loss
- Vomiting and diarrhea
- Seizures or other nervous system disruptions
- Difficulty breathing
- Pain and its management

When symptoms like these become difficult to control, the pet's quality of life is seriously undermined and compromised. It is then appropriate to begin planning in earnest for euthanasia—that is, the peaceful end of the animal's life.

≈

EUTHANASIA: WHEN IT'S TIME
TO SAY GOOD-BYE

The single most difficult aspect of dealing with cancer in a pet is accepting that sometimes cancer shortens a pet's life. Cancer is the *most* treatable and curable chronic disease. Sometimes, however, we can't completely rid the body of disease or the cancer recurs. Treatment options are exhausted or have failed. Hospice care, if the pet has benefited from it, no longer controls pain and prevents suffering. Many of the feelings of helplessness we faced when the cancer was first diagnosed resurface.

Because the cancer patient in this context is an animal, we have the option to choose an end-point to treatment. We can choose to say, "Enough is enough." We can choose (in most cases) when to end the struggle for life, allowing our animal companion to make the transition from this life to the next. Fortunately, we need not make the decision alone. The cancer-fighting team we have assembled—the primary care veterinarian and veterinary nurses, the veterinary cancer specialist and his or her veterinary nurses, the grief counselor, and so on—will help us understand if the time has come to say "Good-bye." They will help us through the decisions, options, and process of *euthanasia.*

What is euthanasia?

Euthanasia is the act of humanely ending an animal's life when that life has become unbearable. The word "euthanasia" comes to us from Greek and means literally "easy death" (*eu* = easy + *thanatos* = death). For the terminally ill animal cancer patient, euthanasia is a gift—a final act of caring. Our focus shifts from "quality of life" to "quality of death." Veterinarians are the only medical professionals empowered to perform euthanasia as part of their practices. The actual procedure of euthanasia is very simple. Death comes quietly and peacefully from an overdose injection of general anesthesia into a vein. Hence the euphemism commonly used for euthanasia—"put to sleep." By using anesthetic agents for this procedure, the animal literally "goes to sleep" and then slips into death.

While the procedure itself is straightforward, the decisions that precede euthanasia are complex, involving many difficult questions that must be answered. The veterinary health care team's objective medical assessments must be combined with our more subjective, intuitive impressions of the pet's quality of life. If we feel that our pet's quality of life is seriously compromised and there is no opportunity for change, then the time has come for the blessing of a smooth passage.

How will I make the decision for euthanasia?

As the pet lives with its cancer, with treatments, and with pain management, its status will be continually evaluated, reevaluated, and assessed. The following questions are usually included in this ongoing evaluation process: Is the pet now in uncontrollable pain? Can the pet control its urine and stool output? Can the pet move about when it chooses to do so? Does the pet recognize the people around it? Is the pet eating and drinking on its own? What about vomiting or diarrhea? Is the pet experiencing uncontrollable seizures or muscle spasms? The veterinary health care team plays a critical role at this point by contributing both objective and subjective clinical impressions and evaluations.

As the pet's human companions, we family members are in the best position to know when the time has come for euthanasia. Our instinctive understanding of our pets helps us know when to stop fighting the cancer. One very important step for the family is to establish, with the help of the veterinary health care team, a personal "bottom line" that defines for us when euthanasia is appropriate. What parameters carry the greatest influence when weighing our decision for euthanasia? How do we define our pet's "quality of life"? What behaviors, postures, breathing patterns, and so on will assist us in knowing the time has come? Setting these standards may relieve some of the anxiety of anticipating the pet's death. We lighten one important burden by establishing benchmarks. Think of this process like establishing a living will for ourselves that defines when life-support measures will be withdrawn in the event of our own illness and impending death.

Once we create our individual "bottom line," cancer demands that we be flexible. Occasionally, a pet will rally unexpectedly. Sometimes our optimistic anticipations are dashed when a pet's attitude and overall demeanor fails more quickly than we have planned. Either way, by thinking ahead, planning ahead, we make the way a little easier for all involved. Once we have listened to input from the veterinary health care team, we must listen to our own hearts and "listen" to our pets, to know when to say good-bye.

Isn't it wrong for me to end my pet's life? Shouldn't I just wait for him to die on his own?

It is easiest for us to accept death—especially death following a long or painful illness—when that death occurs spontaneously, peacefully, and quietly, as during sleep. Unfortunately, death for pets in the home setting is almost never a quiet or peaceful event on its own. When an animal companion is battling an illness like cancer, and is losing that battle, there comes a time when the dignity and quality of life that pet has enjoyed become compromised.

When a person is terminally ill and in the end stages of that illness, we must simply wait for death to come—that is our culture and societal norm. When a pet is in the final stages of illness, however, we are empowered to choose to end the suffering. Pets rarely "die peacefully in their sleep," as most of us would prefer. Instead, most animals must engage in a drawn-out process of failure by stages. Organ systems fail, the ability to control urine and stool outflow fails, the ability to recognize us and the surroundings fails. The pet becomes a shell of the formerly loving and interactive family member it was. In the natural setting (in the wild), a sick cat or dog would never survive very long, for a predator would select the ill animal as prey to kill and eat. Because we shelter and protect our pets as members of the family, they survive to the very end of their ability to hang onto life.

At this difficult time of multilayered failure, we have a most unique gift to offer—the gift of release. Euthanasia is the final gift to the dying. Remember that euthanasia is defined as "easy death." Euthanasia is reserved for that time when simply living is a burden for the pet. When we look into the face of a trusting pet and witness endless pain, the most humane choice we have available is to stop the suffering.

I am feeling overwhelmed at the thought of losing my precious friend after this long and tough battle with cancer. Is it normal that I am so sad already when my pet isn't dead yet?
Although we experience a primary loss at the time the pet dies, many secondary losses occur throughout the course of the disease. Such secondary losses may include a change in the pet's physical appearance, such as the loss of a limb, a change in texture or color of the hair coat, or a change in the pet's appearance from the loss of an eye or part of a jaw. Another secondary loss is a change in the pet's function and activity level. Perhaps he has lost stamina or interest in the usual games he's used to playing. Maybe he simply can't perform at the level of activity he was used to prior to the cancer diagnosis and treatment. The secondary losses we experience may be subtler than the previous examples. Perhaps we feel the effects of an untimely loss of the uniqueness of our relationship with the animal companion. In other words, the bond we forged, the expectations we had for our future with the pet, have changed because of the involvement now of other people in the animal's life as we work through the treatment process.

Secondary losses are stressful. They trigger a phenomenon called *anticipatory grief.* Anticipatory grief leaves us mourning both the lost relationship with the pet, as well as the pet's impending death, no matter if death is expected within days, weeks, or months. Secondary losses are a part of the process. It is absolutely normal to feel sad even before the pet dies.

During cancer treatment, the bond with our pets changes. We become even closer to our animal companions than we ever thought possible. We provide important emotional and physical care and support to the pet. Cancer management and treatment is a long-term process, involving many follow-up visits to the veterinarian for rechecks, treatments, blood evaluations, and so forth. This extra level of bonding may make this particular animal's death more intense than other animal deaths we have experienced before.

We experience grief on many different levels. Normal grieving affects us physically, intellectually, emotionally, and spiritually. It is not important to try to "plan" grief—to try to anticipate all the depths of feeling in which we may be swallowed up. It is important to understand that every person has a unique way of growing through grief.

How does euthanasia happen? What choices will I have?
Ideally, euthanasia involves planning and allows us to have a small measure of control in an otherwise uncontrollable situation. Sometimes, however, the need for euthanasia comes at an unexpected time dictated by sudden changes in the pet's health or level of discomfort. Regardless of the circumstances, you will have choices to make.

The veterinary health care team is ready to assist in that decision-making process.

Decision number one is to determine the location for the euthanasia. More and more, families are choosing to experience the euthanasia of a beloved pet at home. Familiar surroundings and privacy may provide the pet and family with additional comfort at this most painful time. Euthanasia may be performed in the veterinary facility—perhaps in a special area or room that is set apart from the examination rooms. A special room makes the euthanasia feel a bit less clinical, recognizing its deeply personal nature. Each situation is different; each family's preferences are unique. Location details should be worked out among the team members—family and veterinary caregivers.

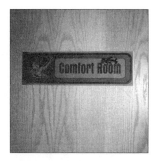

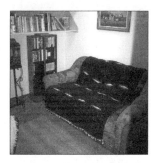

The "Comfort Room" is a special room in the veterinary hospital designed for procedures like euthanasia. It doesn't look or feel like an exam room.

❖

The next decision is whether or not to be present at the time of euthanasia. For some families, it is simply too painful to be present at the moment of death. They prefer to say good-bye in their own way—perhaps with a special treat or meal, or a last walk around the yard—prior to the home euthanasia or to transporting the pet to the

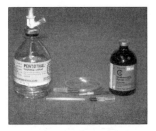

The medications used for euthanasia are delivered directly into a vein to provide a smooth and peaceful transition for the animal.

———— ✛ ————

veterinary hospital. Often, though, families feel encouraged to remain by the pet's side until the moment of death.

Although the details of the procedure may vary slightly from veterinary practice to veterinary practice, euthanasia involves the injection of potent anesthetic drugs that induce a state of deep sleep followed by death. Usually an intravenous catheter is placed in one of the animal's legs first. This ensures that the drugs are delivered directly into the circulation with no risk to the pet of discomfort from an injection that misses the vein. The catheter is a hollow flexible tube designed to rest in the vein and cause no pain. Veterinary health care teams are quite comfortable explaining the details of the euthanasia procedure, so feel free to ask any and all questions that occur to you. They can talk you through every step of the process and ensure that everyone is comfortable with what is happening.

The next decision is how to say good-bye. Sometimes a family will create a short ritual to be carried out at the time of the euthanasia—a special poem or prayer to be recited, snipping some hair to save, making an imprint of the pet's foot in clay—whatever feels most appropriate. Sometimes saying good-bye involves spending a bit of time with the pet's body once the animal has died. The veterinary health care team will do whatever it can to help at this very difficult time.

Should I include my children in the euthanasia event?

Life and death are part of the same cycle. Although including children in the euthanasia event requires some planning and excellent support, it can be an important formative experience for them. Most children who are old enough to think for themselves can participate in the decision making that precedes euthanasia in whatever ways parents feel are appropriate, and they can decide whether or not to be present at the time the animal dies. It is important to be honest with children when a family pet is dying.

The veterinary health care team can assist children who choose to attend the euthanasia of an animal family member. Creating expectations is the key to minimizing trauma and helping children decide how they will say good-bye to an animal friend. If children are to attend euthanasia, they should be told precisely what will happen, what they will see, how the pet will be handled, how the pet will look (Will there be bandages? Will the pet be awake and aware?), what will be appropriate behaviors for them once the animal has died, and so on. Creating expectations is not the same as telling children what to think and feel. Quite the contrary. This approach merely creates structure for the children within which they may safely experience their grief.

Creation of a memorial ceremony or short ritual may be the best way to help a child say good-bye in a healthy fashion. They may want to read a poem or say a prayer for the pet. They may want to cut some hair from the pet's body to save as a memento. Flexibility is important as we help children live with the loss of a best friend.

What do I do with my pet's body?

The veterinary facility that coordinates the pet's cancer treatment program can usually offer several body-handling options. One choice is burial at home. It is best to investigate ahead of time whether there are any local ordinances that dictate animal burial practices—how deep the hole must be, how far away from water or gas lines the grave must be, and so on. Obviously, for those who rent their home, burial is not an appropriate option. Likewise, there are times of the year when burial is simply impossible because of ground conditions—frozen earth is difficult to move even with a back-hoe, and deep mud or a high water table doesn't allow for a deep enough hole.

A second choice is burial at a formal pet cemetery. There are many scattered around the country. Be sure to read the contract carefully to understand how perpetual care is handled. Many pet cemeteries have modeled themselves and their contracts after the human burial business. It is wise to visit the facility and get answers to questions ahead of the pet's death. Few things are more stressful than trying to make important body-handling decisions under the duress of fresh grief.

A third choice for handling a pet's remains is cremation. The crematorium may be at the veterinary hospital, at a pet shelter, or at a business established just for the purpose of pet cremation (with or without burial). Most cremation facilities offer either a "general" or "private" cremation. A general cremation usually means several animal bodies are cremated at once, with the ashes or *cremains* commingled. The crematorium will then usually bury the ashes in a single grave. For a private cremation, the animal's body is alone in the crematorium so that only that pet's ashes remain. The ashes are then collected into an urn or other container and returned to the family. The ashes can then be buried, scattered, or kept, according to the family's wishes.

Another body-handling option is for the remains to be "rendered." This is a high-heat process that extracts usable components from the body for use in

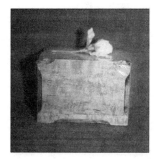

A pet's ashes, following cremation, may be returned in an urn like this one.

———— ✤ ————

glue and other products. Usually, if animal bodies are to be rendered, they are collected and transported by the rendering company with pick up at the veterinary hospital.

Finally, animal bodies may go to a special part of a local landfill where they will deteriorate and become part of the biological environment.

Ironically, the best time for making decisions about a pet's remains is before its death. That gives space, time, and opportunity for adequate planning. By having a plan in place ahead of time, some of the pain of the immediate postdeath period may be eased.

How do my family and I cope with the loss of our "best friend"?
The grief that accompanies the death of a pet can seem overwhelming. One important step in coping is to understand that grief is a process, not an event. It is a very individual experience that happens

on multiple levels—physical, intellectual, emotional, social, and spiritual. Normal grief may last a few days or even years, depending on the nature of the loss. Weeping, nausea, decreased appetite, and changed sleep patterns are quite common during the course of grief, as are an inability to concentrate and "roller coaster" emotions.

Grief over a pet's death will often draw family members together. One classic and still excellent book for understanding and working through the loss of an animal family member is *When Your Pet Dies: How to Cope with Your Feelings* by Jamie Quackenbush, MSW and Denise Graveline. (See the Resources chapter at the end of this book for more recommended reading about pet loss and grief.) You may want to spend time talking with a professional grief counselor—your veterinarian can refer you to qualified individuals in your area.

It is important that everyone in the family has plenty of time and space to work through grief and loss. One good way to memorialize a pet is to have everyone in the family write down on a special sheet of stationery or in a specially chosen blank book who the pet was, what the pet meant to that person, and so on. You may want to include photos or drawings of the pet from different times in its life. You may be tempted to fill the void left by a pet that has died with a new animal addition. Prematurely acquiring a new pet, however, may have just the opposite effect to what is anticipated. Family members will "know" on many levels when the time is right for a new pet to join the family.

How will other animals in my household handle the death of our pet with cancer?

Animals can and do form strong bonds with one another as well as with their human family members. When a family pet dies, it is important to anticipate reactions other animals in the household may have. The other pets may exhibit grief reactions that look remarkably like our own—restlessness, anxiety, changes in sleeping patterns, and so on. Dogs may vocalize inappropriately or incessantly. They may destroy items in the house, or housesoil with urine or stool. The surviving animal may begin to spend more time than usual with the humans in the household.

There are several strategies for assisting surviving pets:

+ Keep daily routines as normal and unchanged as possible. Try to maintain normalcy in the face of loss.
+ Increase playtime with the surviving pet to reward positive behaviors. Increased attention to a pet when it is exhibiting negative behaviors like inappetence or inactivity reinforces unhealthy patterns.
+ Expect a shift in the ways the remaining animals in the household interact with one another. There may be distinct shifts in the social structure. We need to be ready to act as a referee if needed, but it is best for the animals to work out their differences with as little interference as possible.
+ Some families feel that other pets in the household should be present at the euthanasia of an animal family member, although there is no scientific data to suggest that this is essential. This decision is deeply personal, but it may be worthwhile to consider having other animal family members present, especially if the pet with cancer seems to have a particularly close relationship with another pet in the family.

The best approach for surviving pets seems to be keeping household and family routines as normal as possible in the weeks and months following the death of an animal companion. Maintaining a routine may also help the human family members better cope with their own grief.

MURPHY'S STORY

Ironically, though I have had Murphy in my life for the shortest time of all my pets, my bond with her is the strongest. Consequently, I believe that her death will be the most difficult animal death I have yet experienced—both as a veterinarian and as a pet owner.

Because Murphy is such a big dog—150 pounds and very tall—her ability to get up and down and to walk under her own power are important benchmarks in my personal "bottom line." She would be impossible to pick up and carry around. For the same reason—her size—her ability to control her urine and stool output is important. Bone cancer is very painful when it is present in bone itself, so should her cancer recur in her bones, my ability to keep her pain free will weigh heavily in my decision about the timing of her euthanasia. Should her cancer return in her lungs rather than in her bones, it should not be painful for her—in that case, her ability to breathe comfortably will be important.

It is my wish that Murphy's euthanasia will happen at home, in the middle of the living room. I anticipate that our other dogs will be in the house as well. I will hold her big, beautiful head in my lap as the euthanasia drugs take hold and bring her to her final rest, talking to her and reminding her how much I love her. I expect that a trusted colleague will deliver those drugs, for I want to be completely focused on saying good-bye.

Once she is gone, I will have her body cremated and the ashes returned to me. We have an urn, made by a special friend, that contains cremains from other pets we have lost. Murphy's ashes will be added. Because our pets have lived and played together in life, we choose to commingle their ashes in death.

I have made many photos of Murphy during her time with us and continue to do so. We had a professional portrait done of her by a photographer who specializes in pet portraits. I have begun a photo album devoted to her. When I travel to lecture, I often include pictures of Murphy in my talks about pets with cancer—she will travel with me always. No matter when her end comes it will be excruciating, but I am grateful for every day we have together.

Afterword

On 19 September 1999, Murphy celebrated two years of life after cancer treatment. She is active and vital—happy every day to participate in whatever is going on. She goes on a nice long walk nearly every day.

The staff at Windsor Veterinary Clinic threw Murphy a party to celebrate two years cancer-free. Every three months we repeat the recheck procedures, looking for a recurrence of her cancer. So far each recheck has been negative. We continue to hope that she will enjoy a happy, active life for many years to come.

Every day is a gift.

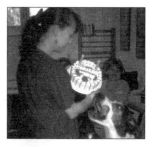

The staff at Windsor Veterinary Clinic threw Murphy a party to celebrate her two-year anniversary of living cancer-free.

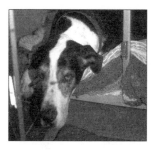

Murphy greets every day with the same upbeat attitude that has sustained her throughout her battle against cancer.

Glossary

acupuncture stimulation of specific points on the body using needles, heat, and so on, for the purpose of balancing energy throughout the body.

anticipatory grief grief we experience *prior* to a pet's death as we anticipate our impending loss.

benign tumors tumors composed of abnormal cells that are not malignant and do not invade or replace normal tissues.

biopsy a representative sample of an abnormal growth that is submitted for analysis and identification.

cancer the general term used to describe the uncontrolled growth of abnormal, invasive cells on or within the body.

cancer cachexia a state of accelerated starvation caused by cancer's takeover of the energy-generating pathways in the body.

cartilage products substances derived from the cartilage of cattle and sharks.

cesium or cobalt therapy another term for radiation therapy.

chemotherapy powerful drugs used to kill cancer cells.

chiropractic medicine a medical treatment using manipulation that focuses on the relationship between the spine and nervous system.

clinical pathologist a veterinary specialist trained to examine, identify, and analyze under the microscope small numbers of cells from a needle biopsy.

complementary therapy medical treatment options that are outside the realm of conventional, accepted, proven treatments.

complete blood count (CBC) evaluation of peripheral blood that assesses bone marrow function by noting the numbers, distribution, and structure of different types of blood cells.

computerized tomography (CT) scan a diagnostic scanning process that uses computer technology to produce images of cross sections through the body.

cremains the ashes that remain after a body has been cremated.

cryosurgery the freezing of tumor cells in a controlled area by applying liquid nitrogen.

debulking the surgical removal of as much of a tumor as possible to decrease the number of tumor cells in the body.

dry or moist desquamation changes in the skin following radiation therapy that resemble sunburn.

endoscopic biopsy a small representative sample of abnormal tissue removed via an endoscope. An endoscope is a thin, flexible tube containing fibers that transmit light. It is used to visualize the inside surfaces of the respiratory system, the digestive system, and the lower urinary tract.

esophagostomy tube a soft rubber feeding tube surgically placed through the side of the neck into the esophagus, maintained to allow food to bypass the mouth.

euthanasia the peaceful ending of a pet's life through the administration of an overdose of anesthesia. Euthanasia is performed when a pet can no longer be kept comfortable.

excisional biopsy removal of an entire tumor with a border of normal tissue on all sides. The "block" of tissue is then submitted for analysis.

fine needle aspirate removal of cells from a tumor by way of a hollow needle and syringe. The cells are then analyzed by a veterinary clinical pathologist. This procedure is also called a needle biopsy.

gastrostomy tube (G-tube) a soft rubber feeding tube surgically placed from the outside of the body directly into the stomach, maintained to allow food to bypass the mouth and esophagus.

grading the process of identifying the level of malignancy of a particular cancer.

herbal and botanical medicine products created from herbs and other plants that are used for medical purposes.

histopathologist another term for surgical pathologist.

homeopathic medicine a treatment option involving very dilute remedies made from naturally occurring substances.

hospice care compassionate care administered to an animal patient prior to euthanasia but after cancer therapy stops working.

hypercalcemia abnormally elevated levels of calcium in the blood.

immune modulation therapy stimulation of the immune system in very specific ways to assist in killing cancer cells.

immunoaugmentive therapy an experimental cancer treatment that involves injecting blood products daily into the animal patient for the purpose of stimulating the pet's immune system.

incisional biopsy removal of a representative sample of a tumor via a surgical incision.

irradiation another term for radiation therapy.

jejunostomy tube (J-tube) a soft rubber feeding tube surgically placed directly into the small intestine, maintained to allow food to bypass the mouth, esophagus, and stomach.

magnetic resonance imaging (MRI) a computer-assisted imaging technology especially well suited for uncovering tumors in the soft tissues of the body.

malignant tumors tumors that invade other tissues or destroy and replace normal cells.

mass another term for tumor.

massage therapy medical treatment that involves manipulation of body tissues with a focus on muscles, circulation, and the nervous system.

meridians parallel channels of energy that flow throughout the body and are modified with the application of acupuncture.

metastasis the relocation and growth of cancer cells from the original tumor site to other parts of the body.

mucositis a side effect of radiation therapy in which the mucous membranes that line the mouth develop irritation and ulceration. Mucositis is a temporary event.

multifocal a term used to indicate that disease is present in more than one location in the body.

nasogastric tube (N-G tube) a small-diameter, soft rubber tube that is passed through a nostril, through the nasal passages, and down the esophagus into the stomach for delivery of liquid nutrients, bypassing the mouth.

needle biopsy removal of cells from a tumor by way of a hollow needle and syringe. The cells are then analyzed by a veterinary clinical pathologist. This procedure is also called fine needle aspirate.

nutritional therapy the use of specific nutrients or lifestyle diets to treat disease.

orthovoltage therapy another term for radiation therapy.

osteosarcoma a type of cancer originating in bone.

ovariohysterectomy surgical removal of the uterus and ovaries from the female animal.

palliative treatment (e.g., palliative radiation) any treatment used for the purpose of relieving symptoms associated with a tumor rather than with the intention of curing the cancer.

paraneoplastic event or syndrome a symptom or set of symptoms that result from cancer, but which are felt in the body far from the original tumor site.

pharmacological and biological therapy treatment options involving drugs, vaccines, or other materials (e.g., shark cartilage) not yet accepted by the traditional medical establishment.

preemptive pain management medicating to prevent pain and discomfort.

radiation therapy the application of specific, intense energy from a machine or radioactive substance that can kill cancer cells or prevent them from growing and dividing.

radiograph the image produced on special film when X rays are passed through a part of the body. The X rays are blocked to varying degrees by the tissues of the body, producing many shades of gray on the radiograph. Denser tissues like bone block more X rays and appear white, soft tissues like muscle block fewer X rays and appear gray, and air blocks no X rays and appears black.

radiotherapy another term for radiation therapy.

recurrence return of cancer after it has been treated.

remission the period of time during which cancer is inactive following treatment.

serum biochemical profile blood tests that evaluate organ system functions, blood sugar, and levels of minerals in the body.

squamous cell carcinoma a type of cancer originating in the skin.

surgical pathologist (histopathologist) a veterinary pathologist trained to identify and evaluate fixed, stained samples of tissue under the microscope.

total parenteral nutrition (TNP) a method of providing all necessary nutrients intravenously.

tumor group of abnormal cells growing in an organized structure.

tumor margin the border around a tumor's outer perimeter that is carefully evaluated by the surgical pathologist to determine if all cancer cells have been removed at surgery.

urinalysis evaluation of the components of urine, including a microscopic examination of any cellular debris.

X-ray therapy another term for radiation therapy.

Resources

Additional Resources and Reading

The Affection Connection, Will the Sadness Go Away? Manhattan, KS: Cooperative Extension Service, Kansas State University, 1991.
This videotape is designed for use by veterinarians, parents, and teachers. To order, call Kansas State University Research and Extension Distribution Center, 785-532-5830, and ask for videotape SV286.

Boulden, J. *Saying Good-Bye Activity Book*. Santa Rosa, CA: Jim Boulden Publications, 1989.
A coloring and activity book that encourages children to explore their feelings about death. To order, contact Boulden Publishing, PO Box 1186, Weaverville, CA 96093; 800-238-8433.

Brackenridge, S. *Because of Flowers and Dancers*. Santa Barbara, CA: Veterinary Practice Publishing Company, 1994.

Buscaglia, L. *The Fall of Freddie the Leaf: A Story for All Ages*. New York: Slack Book Division, 1982.

Fine, J. *Afraid to Ask: A Book for Families to Share about Cancer*. New York: Beach Tree Books, 1986.

Morehead, D. *A Special Place for Charlee: A Child's Companion through Pet Loss.* Broomfield, CO: Partners in Publishing, 1996.

Quackenbush, J. and Graveline, D. *When Your Pet Dies: How to Cope with Your Feelings.* New York: Pocket Books (Simon & Schuster), 1985.

Rogers, F. *When a Pet Dies.* New York: Putnam Publishing Group, 1988.

Rylant, C. *Cat Heaven.* New York: Blue Sky Press, 1997.

Rylant, C. *Dog Heaven.* New York: Blue Sky Press, 1995.

Viorst, J. *The Tenth Good Thing about Barney.* New York: Aladdin Books, 1988.

Wilhelm, H. *I'll Always Love You.* New York: Crown Publishers, 1985.

Websites of Interest

American Animal Hospital Association Healthy Pets Web Page
www.healthypet.com
The American Animal Hospital Association is an organization of over 17,000 veterinary care providers committed to excellence in small animal care. This website can provide you with information about helping your pet be healthy, as well as assist you in a search for a veterinary health care provider.

American Veterinary Medical Association Care for Pets Web Page
www.avma.org/care4pets
This website offers great general information about pets, pet health care, pet safety, and veterinarians.

Bacup
www.bacup.or.uk/index.shtml
This is a terrific human cancer website recognized as the foremost provider of cancer information in the United Kingdom.

CancerNet™—National Cancer Institute Website
cancernet.nci.nih.gov
Sponsored by the National Cancer Institute, CancerNet™ is a website that will connect you to a wide range of human cancer information.

Guide to Internet Resources for Cancer
www.ncl.ac.uk/%7Encbwww/guides/clinks1.htm
This human cancer website is also based in the United Kingdom.

Hill's® Pet Nutrition Website
www.hillspet.com
Hill's® Pet Nutrition, Inc., manufactures specialty and maintenance foods for pets, including Prescription Diet® Canine n/d®, the diet formulated to support dogs with cancer.

Miscellaneous Human Cancer Related Links
seidata.com/%7Emarriage/rcancer.html
This website provides links to many human cancer websites.

North Carolina Animal Cancer Treatment Program
www2.ncsu.edu/ncsu/cvm/VTH/oncol.html
This website provides news about animal cancer work ongoing at North Carolina State University College of Veterinary Medicine.

The Veterinary Cancer Society Website
vetcancersociety.org
The Veterinary Cancer Society is a nonprofit educational organization dedicated to maintaining the highest standards of treatment and prevention of cancer in animals. Here you will find answers to frequently asked questions, information about cancer in animals, and links to related sites.

Veterinary Teaching Hospitals in the United States and Canada
Colleges of veterinary medicine and their affiliated veterinary teaching hospitals provide access to specially trained individuals as well as specialized diagnostic and treatment options for pets.

Auburn University, College of Veterinary Medicine, Auburn University, AL 36849; Main Telephone Number: 334-844-4546.

University of California, School of Veterinary Medicine, Davis, CA 95616-8734; Main Telephone Number: 916-752-1360.

Colorado State University, College of Veterinary Medicine and Biological Sciences, Ft. Collins, CO 80523; Main Telephone Number: 970-491-7051.

Cornell University, College of Veterinary Medicine, Ithaca, NY 14853-6401; Main Telephone Number: 607-253-4072.

University of Florida, College of Veterinary Medicine, Gainesville, FL 32610-0125; Main Telephone Number: 352-392-4700, ext. 5000.

University of Georgia, College of Veterinary Medicine, Athens, GA 30602; Main Telephone Number: 706-542-3461.

University of Illinois, College of Veterinary Medicine, 2001 South Lincoln, Urbana, IL 61801; Main Telephone Number: 217-333-2760.

Iowa State University, College of Veterinary Medicine, Ames, IA 50011; Main Telephone Number: 515-294-1242.

Kansas State University, College of Veterinary Medicine, Manhattan, KS 66506; Main Telephone Number: 913-532-5660.

Louisiana State University, School of Veterinary Medicine, Baton Rouge, LA 70803; Main Telephone Number: 504-346-3100.

Michigan State University, College of Veterinary Medicine, East Lansing, MI 48824-1314; Main Telephone Number: 517-355-6509.

University of Minnesota, College of Veterinary Medicine, St. Paul, MN 55108; Main Telephone Number: 612-624-9927.

Mississippi State University, College of Veterinary Medicine, Mississippi State, MI 39762; Main Telephone Number: 601-325-3432.

University of Missouri, College of Veterinary Medicine, Columbia, MO 65211; Main Telephone Number: 573-882-3877.

University of Montreal, Faculty of Veterinary Medicine, Saint Hyacinthe, Quebec, Canada J2S 7C6; Main Telephone Number: 514-345-8521.

North Carolina State University, College of Veterinary Medicine, 4700 Hillsborough Street, Raleigh, NC 27606; Main Telephone Number: 919-829-4210.

Ohio State University, College of Veterinary Medicine, Columbus, OH 43210; Main Telephone Number: 614-292-1171.

Oklahoma State University, College of Veterinary Medicine, Stillwater, OK 74078; Main Telephone Number: 405-744-6648.

Ontario Veterinary College, University of Guelph, Guelph, Ontario, Canada N1G 2W1; Main Telephone Number: 519-823-8800, ext. 4417.

College of Veterinary Medicine at Oregon State University, Corvallis, OR 97331; Main Telephone Number: 541-737-2141.

University of Pennsylvania, School of Veterinary Medicine, 3800 Spruce Street, Philadelphia, PA 19104-6044; Main Telephone Number: 215-898-5438.

University of Prince Edward Island, Atlantic Veterinary College, Charlottetown, Prince Edward Island, Canada C1A 4P3; Main Telephone Number: 902-566-0800.

Purdue University, School of Veterinary Medicine, 1240 Lynn Hall, West Lafayette, IN 47907-1240; Main Telephone Number: 765-494-7607.

University of Saskatchewan, Western College of Veterinary Medicine, 52 Campus Drive, Saskatoon, Saskatchewan, Canada S7N 5B4; Main Telephone Number: 306-966-7448.

University of Tennessee, College of Veterinary Medicine, Knoxville, TN 37901; Main Telephone Number: 423-974-7262.

Texas A & M University, College of Veterinary Medicine, College Station, TX 77843-4461; Main Telephone Number: 409-845-5051.

Tufts University, School of Veterinary Medicine, 200 Westboro Road, North Grafton, MA 01536; Main Telephone Number: 508-839-5302.

Tuskegee University, School of Veterinary Medicine, Tuskegee, AL 36088; Main Telephone Number: 334-727-8174.

Virginia Tech and University of Maryland, Virginia-Maryland Regional College of Veterinary Medicine, Blacksburg, VA 24061-0442; Main Telephone Number: 540-231-7666.

Washington State University, College of Veterinary Medicine, Pullman, WA 99164-7010; Main Telephone Number: 509-335-9515.

University of Wisconsin-Madison, School of Veterinary Medicine, Madison, WI 53706; Main Telephone Number: 608-263-6716.

Bibliography

Clough, E., and J. Clough. "Helping Clients Say Good-bye: A Hospice Service for Pets," in *Proceedings for FasTrack to a Better Practice*. Baltimore, MD: Annual Convention of the AVMA, 1998.

Cohen, S. P., and C. E. Fudin, eds. "Animal Illness and Human Emotion." *Problems in Veterinary Medicine*, 3, no. 1 (March 1991).

Couto, G. C. "Cancer Management," in *The Veterinary CE Advisor* (a supplement to *Veterinary Medicine*). Lenexa, KS: Veterinary Medicine Publishing Group, 1998.

Couto, C. G. "Cancer Therapy: Evaluating Options." *Veterinary Technician* 18, no. 8 (1997): 553-563.

Couto, C. G. "Oncology," in *Small Animal Internal Medicine*, 2nd ed., ed. R. W. Nelson, C. G. Couto, 1092-1157. St. Louis, MO: Mosby, 1998.

Couto, G. C., Guest Editor. "Clinical Management of the Cancer Patient." *The Veterinary Clinics of North America: Small Animal Practice* 20, no. 4 (July 1990).

Crow, S. E. "Managing Cancer: Early Diagnosis by Primary Care DVMs Critical to Success. *DVM Newsmagazine* (November 1997): 5-6S.

Crow, S. E. "Set Realistic Treatment Goals for Patients, Owners." *DVM Newsmagazine* (December 1997): 1-3S.

Davenport, D. J., and G. K. Ogilvie. *Canine Cancer: Management of Canine Cancer.* Topeka, KS: Hill's® Pet Nutrition, 1998.

DiLima, S. N., and L. Stock, eds. *Oncology Patient Education Manual.* An Aspen Publication. Aspen Reference Group. Gaithersburg, MD: Aspen Publishers, 1997.

Fine, J. *Afraid to Ask: A Book for Families to Share about Cancer.* New York: Beach Tree Books, 1986.

Gilson, S. D., Guest Editor. "Surgical Oncology." *The Veterinary Clinics of North America: Small Animal Practice* 25, no. 1 (January 1995).

Hammond, A. "Dealing with Grief in Relation to Companion Animals and Cancer," in *Proceedings 224, Treatment of Cancer in Companion Animals,* 235–249. Sydney, Australia: University of Sydney, Post-Graduate Committee in Veterinary Science, 1994.

Klein, M. K., and W. G. Roberts. "Recent Advances in Photodynamic Therapy." *Compendium on Continuing Education for the Practicing Veterinarian* 15, no. 6 (1993): 809–818.

Lagoni, L. *The Practical Guide to Client Grief.* Denver, CO: AAHA Press, 1997.

Lagoni, L., C. Butler, and S. Hetts. *The Human-Animal Bond and Grief.* Philadelphia, PA: W. B. Saunders, 1994.

LaRue, S. M., and E. L. Gillette. "Recent Advances in Radiation Oncology." *Compendium on Continuing Education for the Practicing Veterinarian* 15, no. 6 (1993): 795–805.

MacEwen, E. G. "The Pet with Cancer: Impact on the Family," in *Euthanasia of the Companion Animal*, ed. W. J. Kay, 97–100. Philadelphia, PA: The Charles Press, 1988.

MacEwen, E. G., and S. C. Helfand. "Recent Advances in the Biologic Therapy of Cancer." *Compendium on Continuing Education for the Practicing Veterinarian* 15, no. 7 (1993): 909–923.

Morrison, W. B. *Cancer in Dogs and Cats: Medical and Surgical Management.* Baltimore, MD: Williams and Wilkins, 1998.

O'Brien, M. G., R. C. Straw, and S. J. Withrow. "Recent Advances in the Treatment of Canine Appendicular Osteosarcoma." *Compendium on Continuing Education for the Practicing Veterinarian* 15, no. 7 (1993): 939–948.

Ogilvie, G. K. "Alterations in Metabolism and Nutritional Support for Veterinary Cancer Patients: Recent Advances." *Compendium on Continuing Education for the Practicing Veterinarian* 15, no. 7 (1993): 925–937.

Ogilvie, G. K., and A. S. Moore. *Managing the Veterinary Cancer Patient*. Trenton, New Jersey: Veterinary Learning Systems Company, 1995.

Ogilvie, G. K., and N. G. Robinson. "Complementary/Alternative Cancer Therapy—Fact or Fiction?" in *Textbook of Veterinary Internal Medicine*, 4th ed., ed. S. E. Ettinger. Philadelphia, PA: W. B. Saunders, 1999.

Page, R. L. "Recent Advances in Hyperthermia." *Compendium on Continuing Education for the Practicing Veterinarian* 15, no. 6 (1993): 781–792.

Quackenbush, J., and D. Graveline. *When Your Pet Dies: How to Cope with Your Feelings*. New York: Pocket Books (Simon & Schuster), 1985.

Ruslander, D. "Client Counseling for Owners of Cancer Patients," in *Proceedings of Small Animal Oncology Conference*. Zurich, Switzerland: University of Zurich, 1998.

Withrow, S. J., and E. G. MacEwen. *Small Animal Clinical Oncology*. Philadelphia, PA: W. B. Saunders, 1996.

Index

Note: Italicized page numbers indicate photos.

About the Author

Since graduating from the College of Veterinary Medicine at the University of Illinois at Champaign-Urbana in 1986, Dr. Downing has been blazing her own trail within veterinary medicine as well as her community.

As the first (and only) woman veterinarian for a 100-mile radius in Worland, Wyoming, from 1986 to 1991, Dr. Downing brought sophisticated companion animal medicine into the homes of pet lovers. She built a successful veterinary practice in an economically challenged area, learning important life-lessons along the way. She was the 1988 National Federation of Business and Professional Women's Outstanding Young Career Woman for the state of Wyoming.

In 1991, Dr. Downing purchased Windsor Veterinary Clinic, a stagnant practice in small-town Colorado. Achieving four-year accreditation status with the American Animal Hospital Association in 1994, Windsor Veterinary Clinic, PC, was named one of the first 10 Practice of Excellence Award® winners in the United States that same year. Her practice was featured in the January 1995 issue of *Veterinary Economics Magazine*.

In addition to creating an award-winning practice, Dr. Downing is committed to personal excellence. She was the 1995 Colorado Veterinary Medical Association's Up and Coming Veterinarian of the Year, and the 1996 Association for Women Veterinarians' Outstanding

Woman Veterinarian of the Year. In 1999 she received a regional Entrepreneurial Excellence Award® from *Working Woman Magazine*, and has been named the Hill's Animal Welfare and Humane Ethics Award winner for the year 2000.

Dr. Downing passionately shares her vision for the bright future of veterinary medicine with audiences of every ilk. She has participated in many major veterinary conferences, as well as many state and local meetings. She and her business/life partner, Sharon DeNayer, presented First Line Live!®, an innovative training for the veterinary support team, at several locations in 1997, 1998, and 1999. Dr. Downing is an outspoken advocate of the precious nature of the Family-Pet Bond when the pet faces special challenges like chronic illness, cancer, or a physical disability. She was delighted to present this topic to a pet-loving audience at the Smithsonian Institution in Washington, D.C., in 1997.

Putting to good use her English degree from Loyola University of Chicago, Dr. Downing is a respected author on animal-related issues. She is a regular contributing author to *Veterinary Economics Magazine*, and serves on the Editorial Advisory Board of *Veterinary Economics*. Dr. Downing is a featured weekly columnist in the *Sunday Denver Post*, answering the questions of concerned pet owners. She authored a selection in *Chicken Soup for the Pet Lover's Soul*.

An accomplished old-time fiddler, she has numerous trophies from competition at the Wyoming State Old-time Fiddle Contest. Dr. Downing shares her home with eleven cats, five dogs, two birds, a ferret, and a squirrel — all cast-offs, slated for euthanasia or abandonment — all thriving within a microcosm of unconditional love.